Acupu̶   ̶ Practice

Beyond points and meridians

Dedication

For Marie-Christine, whose organizational flair has been essential to the acupuncture courses from which this book has developed.

Senior commissioning editor: Heidi Allen
Development editor: Robert Edwards
Production controller: Anthony Read
Desk editor: Jackie Holding
Cover design: Gregory Harris

Acupuncture in Practice

Beyond points and meridians

Anthony Campbell MRCP(UK), Dip. Med. Ac., F.F. Hom.,
Emeritus Consultant Physician, Royal London Homeopathic Hospital

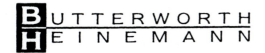

OXFORD   AUCKLAND   BOSTON   JOHANNESBURG   MELBOURNE   NEW DELHI

BUTTERWORTH-HEINEMANN
An imprint of Elsevier Limited

First published 2001
Reprinted 2003 (twice), 2005

British Library Cataloguing in Publication Data
A catalogue record for this book is available from the British Library

Library of Congress Cataloguing in Publication Data
A catalogue record for this book is available from the Library of Congress

ISBN 0 7506 5242 X

Transferred to digital printing 2006

Contents

Acknowledgements

I should like to thank Heidi Allen, Robert Edwards, Jackie Holding, and the rest of the team at Butterworth-Heinemann for the care and interest they have taken in the production of this book.

Foreword

Acupuncture is full of controversies, and none is greater than the fundamental approach we should adopt. On the one hand, the traditional practice of acupuncture has evolved over many centuries of clinical observation and been passed down by respected masters to grateful apprentices. Supporters of the traditional approach argue that its concepts of energy flow operate as a knowledge system in its own right which should not be rejected just because it does not fit in with current western understanding of the body's mechanisms. On the other hand, the 'modern' approach declares that acupuncture is a relatively straightforward form of stimulation therapy that is beginning to be explained in physiological terms. So, learning complicated rules about where to place the needles and different methods of stimulating them is no longer necessary.

This debate is particularly active in Britain, where Anthony Campbell is perhaps the best known proponent of the modern approach, and certainly the most articulate. He was originally attracted to acupuncture by his knowledge of and fascination for eastern philosophy. He soon came across Felix Mann, one of the first to challenge the old ideas and look afresh at what happens when a patient is needled. Anthony was instinctively sympathetic to a modern approach, and tested it carefully by many years of careful observation of his own patients. Through teaching, the rigour of his thinking has been refined in the hot fire of critical challenge by students. He has been prepared to knock down (but always politely: he is highly respectful of traditional philosophies in themselves) any icons or preconceptions that are not common sense and that hinder progress. The sum of all this wisdom and experience is accumulated in this text, which will stand as one of the most thoughtful yet accessible treatises on acupuncture of all time.

This is a radical book that succeeds in demystifying acupuncture. It presents a closely argued but entirely practical approach to needling patients. It is compatible with the little we do know about the function of the nervous system, requiring no leap of faith or suspension of disbelief. Anthony Campbell does not claim to provide short-cut recipes for treating patients – that still requires careful thought and application of basic principles. He accepts that there are plenty of aspects of acupuncture that we still cannot explain, but reassures the reader that modern science is the best way of finding useful and meaningful answers. This book reflects the author's truly innovative contributions in certain particular aspects of the technique, most notably what he calls the 'acupuncture treatment areas' that replace traditional points. He also emphasizes the likely role of the brain's limbic system, which suggests that patients' nervous systems must in some way be 'prepared' (but not simply by suggestion or belief) if acupuncture is to be really successful, which in turn leads on to an open acceptance of the essential role of 'placebo' in all clinical practice. This book promises to become a milestone in the debate about acupuncture and the development of a rational approach to the technique.

Adrian White

Preface

Acupuncture has been known in the West for about 400 years. Although initially greeted with puzzlement, it attracted the attention of some Western physicians, and at times, particularly in the nineteenth century, it was used quite extensively. The main difference today is that interest in acupuncture is part of a wider enthusiasm for complementary and alternative medicine (CAM), and this has prompted a large number of health professionals (doctors, physiotherapists, osteopaths, chiropractors, podiatrists, for example) to wish to learn acupuncture in order to help their patients. They tend, however, to be discouraged by two preconceptions. One is that studying the traditional system is difficult and time-consuming, and the other is that treating patients in this way is itself time-consuming (most Western practitioners of traditional acupuncture leave the needles in place for 20 minutes or more).

However, there is now a considerable amount of clinical experience in the West, supported by some research, to show that neither of these ideas is necessarily true. The elaborate traditional theory, though doubtless of great historical and cultural interest, does not appear to be essential in practice. It is possible to simplify the techniques considerably without sacrificing their clinical effectiveness. If acupuncture is approached as a form of peripheral stimulation of the nervous system it becomes much more accessible to people trained in modern anatomy and physiology. Many of us have also found that prolonged insertion of needles is unnecessary; in almost all cases brief insertion, lasting a few minutes or even a few seconds, is all that is required. It is therefore perfectly possible to fit acupuncture into a busy treatment schedule.

Most of what is written about acupuncture still approaches the subject from the traditional aspect and there is relatively little available about the modern version. In consequence, many health professionals do not even realize that anything other than traditional acupuncture exists, and still less do they understand the practical advantages of studying acupuncture in the modern way. In this book I explain what modern acupuncture is and how it can be applied in practice. The book is not intended to be a substitute for hands-on instruction, for acupuncture can't be learned from books, but it will provide the knowledge and understanding needed by anyone who is considering undertaking practical tuition of this kind. It is the textbook which I use on my own courses for health professionals.

Introduction

Acupuncture is a method of treating certain disorders by inserting needles into various parts of the body. Its value is that it works in some disorders for which there is little or no effective treatment and that, in competent hands, it is relatively safe.

Acupuncture developed in China, where it acquired an elaborate theoretical basis. Recently it has been taken up by a number of Western health professionals, many of whom have reinterpreted it in terms of modern anatomy, physiology and pathology. Today, therefore, there exist two main schools of acupuncture, traditional and modern.

The principal differences between the traditional and modern schools can be summarized as follows:

Traditional	Modern
Follows rules laid down in the past	Largely ignores the old rules
Based on prescientific ideas	Based on modern anatomy and physiology
Practical rather than mystical but appeals to Westerners interested in mysticism	No element of mysticism

The chief advantage of the modern approach, so far as Westerners are concerned, is that it can be assimilated easily into the rest of medical training. Also, it has given rise to some new forms of treatment, such as periosteal acupuncture, that did not form part of the traditional system.

Learning acupuncture in its traditional form is a lengthy process, a fact which often leads to demands for hundreds of hours of training. The essentials of modern acupuncture, in contrast, can be grasped in much less time. In fact, I start from the position that acquiring basic acupuncture skills is easy. This probably surprising statement is based on certain assumptions, the main one being that you are a conventionally trained Western health professional. If you are, you already possess, without realizing it, most of the skill and knowledge you need to practise acupuncture; all you have to do is to learn to apply them in a different context. You are, in fact, in the position of Molière's Monsieur Jourdain, who found that he had been speaking prose all his life without realizing it.

By 'health professional', I mean, for example, a doctor, physiotherapist, osteopath, chiropractor, hand therapist, podiatrist, or nurse working in pain clinics and similar environments, all of whom have acquired knowledge of anatomy and physiology and are used to working as clinicians. Naturally, not all these professionals will have the same requirements or use acupuncture in the same way, but all can apply acupuncture to some extent in their practice.

I wish to demystify acupuncture. By definition, the treatment consists in the insertion of needles, but there is nothing distinctive about the use of needles themselves; they are merely one effective means of stimulating the peripheral nervous system. Pressing the tissues or burning them may have similar effects; 'acupressure' and moxibustion are applications of this principle. Other stimuli could be applied as well, and the mechanism of action of acupuncture is probably similar to that of manual physiotherapy, osteopathy, chiropractic, and even massage. All these forms of therapy seem to act by modifying central nervous system processing, and there is a lot of overlapping among all the manual techniques. This idea makes acupuncture easier to assimilate to existing therapies.

If acupuncture is approached in the way I suggest here, it becomes a technique, or set of techniques, much like any other. But please understand that this isn't an oversimplified version, suitable only for people too lazy or too set in their ways to study 'real' acupuncture in its traditional form; it doesn't, I hope, sacrifice anything worth keeping. On the contrary, it is, I believe, the most effective way of doing acupuncture, because what is unnecessary and confusing has been removed, leaving the essential core of the procedure intact. I don't claim any great originality for my approach, nor do I deny that there are other ways of doing acupuncture that also work, but I do claim to have cut away a good deal of dead wood. Changing the metaphor, what I have tried to do is to distil, from the complex brew of acupuncture fact and fiction, a concentrated version that preserves the essence of the treatment and makes it available to any health professional.

The plan of the book is as follows. In Part 1 I look at the differences between traditional and modern acupuncture and point out some commonly held misconceptions about what the traditional system actually is, or was. Finally, I define what I mean by modern acupuncture and try to provide at least a tentative explanation for how it may work in the relief of pain.

Part 2 is the core of the book, which contains what I take to be the essence of modern acupuncture. Here I first review the safety aspects of acupuncture, which everyone intending to practise these techniques must be familiar with. I then look at the different ways of deciding where to insert the needles that are currently in vogue in modern acupuncture. Each of these has its merits, but the fact that there are so many such ways is likely to confuse the newcomer to acupuncture. I therefore put forward my own version, based on what I call the Acupuncture Treatment Area (ATA). My aim is to equip the reader with a way of thinking about acupuncture that will free him or her from dependence on theory and allow a more creative approach to treatment. This approach has emerged from many years' experience of teaching the subject to health professionals.

Part 3 shows how the ideas set forth in Part 2 can be applied in practice. To do this I go through the various anatomical regions (head and neck, thorax, lower back, and so on), describing the acupuncture treatments that can be used in each and the kinds of effects that can be expected. This section is not intended to be a 'cookbook' – a set of rules about what to do in each situation. On the contrary, I want to guide the reader away from the cookbook method. The descriptions of treatments are meant to be illustrations of the principles discussed earlier, not a list of prescriptions.

Plain descriptions of techniques and treatments are liable to make dry reading, so I have included a number of case histories for the sake of variety and illustration. They are not, of course, intended to provide supportive evidence for my arguments or for the effectiveness of the treatments I describe. Such evidence can come only from scientific research, which at present is sadly lacking for most claims made on behalf of acupuncture. I look at some of the manifold problems of acupuncture research in Part 4, where I also write about some specialized forms of acupuncture, such as auriculotherapy, and consider the uses of electricity in acupuncture.

It isn't essential to read the book from cover to cover. Readers with no interest in the traditional system, and who are already sure that it's the modern version of acupuncture that appeals to them, could go directly to the practical sections. If you do this, however, please read Part 2, otherwise the reasons for choosing the treatments described in Part 3 won't be evident to you.

Part 1

Chapter 1

Ancient or modern?

This is a book about modern acupuncture. To some, this statement may sound like a contradiction in terms. Isn't acupuncture a system of vast antiquity that developed in China many thousands of years ago? Well, yes, it is that, but in the last few decades there has come into being a different way of thinking about the treatment, based on modern ideas of anatomy, physiology, and the nature of disease instead of on yin and yang. The modern version of acupuncture is the kind that I practise and teach to health professionals in short courses. This is, admittedly, a somewhat contentious matter, for some people maintain that the only 'real' acupuncture is the traditional version, which requires months or even years of study to master. (An eloquent defence of this position has been mounted by Richard James, a Western doctor trained in the traditional system (James, 1998).) Nothing useful can be achieved in a short course, traditionalists aver, or at most the practitioner may learn to treat some 'simple' disorders that don't require the sophisticated and subtle understanding possessed by the authentic Chinese practitioner. However, I am unrepentant. I maintain that modern acupuncture can be every bit as effective as the traditional version, and indeed it offers certain forms of treatment, such as periosteal acupuncture, that didn't form part of the traditional version but which give better results in certain circumstances. These are opinions arrived at in the light of experience. And yet, before I actually learned acupuncture myself, I had quite different expectations and assumptions.

I started practising acupuncture in 1977, shortly after I had begun working as a consultant at the Royal London Homeopathic Hospital. This is a National Health Service hospital that was founded, over a hundred years ago, to provide homeopathy. Nowadays, however, it's a centre specializing in a number of complementary therapies in addition to homeopathy, and moreover all the staff have a background and qualifications in conventional medicine or therapeutics as well.

I had originally had no intention of practising the modern type of acupuncture; indeed, I didn't know that such a thing existed. I had been interested in acupuncture, and in Chinese and Indian ideas generally, for a number of years before encountering acupuncture in a practical sense. I had read a fair amount of Taoist literature in translation and found it both appealing and fascinating, so I was well-disposed towards traditional Chinese medicine and assumed, as a matter of course, that if one wanted to learn acupuncture one would have to go about it in the traditional way. At first I knew of no way to do this, but then I heard that a doctor, Felix Mann, taught acupuncture. I enrolled for a five-day course. Before the course we were asked to read some of the books he'd written, which at that time were entirely about the traditional system. I did so, with a good deal of bewilderment. I realized acupuncture might be difficult but this was worse than I expected; all this talk of meridians, points, pulses and whatnot seemed impossibly complicated and more alien even than homeopathy had been at the outset. It was thus with some trepidation that I presented myself at Felix's house in Devonshire Place to start the course.

There were fourteen of us. We sat on rather hard chairs in a semicircle while Felix sat in the middle and talked to us; at intervals during the week patients came to tell us their stories and receive their treatment. The first thing Felix told us was that he did not believe in the traditional apparatus of meridians, acupuncture points and so on. We were naturally taken aback by this and asked him why, in that case, he had told us to read his books. He replied that it was necessary to be familiar with the traditional stuff in order to leave it behind. He then explained why he no longer believed it. When he started out in acupuncture, he said, he did do it in the traditional way, but then he tried doing it in the 'wrong' way, ignoring the traditional theory and putting the needles in 'incorrect' places, and found that the results were just as good. He therefore concluded that the ancient theory, though it might be founded on accurate observations, was mistaken.

I have to admit that my initial feeling was one of disappointment. As I have said, it was largely because of my fascination with Taoism and Chinese philosophy in general that I had wanted to study acupuncture, and it was something of a letdown to be told that the traditional theory wasn't valid and that acupuncture could work just as well or even better if one ignored it. On the other hand, it was definitely a relief not to have to learn all this complicated stuff, and I respected Felix's intellectual honesty in abandoning it when he found that it didn't seem to be valid. As the course went on and the patients kept coming and telling their stories, I was impressed by what I was seeing and hearing; Felix's attitude to acupuncture was practical and down-to-earth and the patients certainly seemed to be responding well. But would it work for me? There was only one way to find out.

As soon as I returned from the course I started to try out what I had learnt. I set aside a clinic to do acupuncture, though at this stage I didn't designate it formally as such. My first patient was a young woman who had suffered a whiplash injury in a car accident about a year previously.

For the past year she had been attending a medical osteopath in Harley Street who was well known at the time but is now dead. The patient still had a lot of pain in her neck and didn't feel she had been helped. I offered her acupuncture and she accepted. Trying to look and sound more confident than I felt, I needled her neck in the way I had seen Felix do it. All seemed to go quite well in the short term and I asked her to return in a couple of weeks' time. She did so, and reported that she was much better. I repeated the treatment on a few more occasions and soon she was symptom-free. I saw her on and off over the years that followed and she always did well with acupuncture, but not until almost twenty years later did I summon up the courage to tell her that she had been the first patient I ever treated with the needles. (She took it very well, I'm glad to say!)

Perhaps, I thought, this was beginner's luck. However, I continued to treat patients, and many did well. The success rate with acupuncture was about 70 per cent. Moreover, the results were reasonably predictable – not in every case, of course, but in general. When I saw a new patient with backache, perhaps, or headaches, I could say reasonably confidently that the chances of getting a fair degree of improvement were pretty good. Naturally my results improved as my experience and manual dexterity with the needles got better, but from the beginning I found that I was getting worthwhile results. I felt encouraged to persevere with acupuncture and, some years later, to start my own courses for teaching it to doctors and other health professionals. Most of the doctors at the hospital came on these courses, and eventually a large amount of acupuncture was carried out there: about 500 treatments a week, for a wide variety of disorders.

How I see acupuncture today

Because I was initially attracted to acupuncture through a longstanding interest in Far Eastern ideas, I can understand why others feel drawn towards traditional acupuncture. I have, nevertheless, come to believe that it's best to separate any interest one may have in ancient Chinese ideas from the practical aspects of acupuncture. Read about the Tao, yin and yang, and the rest of it by all means – there is much to be gained from immersing oneself for a time in an ancient and alien way of thought – but come back to the present and to science when you pick up the needles.

I know that this is an unwelcome message for some. The esoteric aspects of traditional acupuncture constitute much of its appeal for quite a number of practitioners (and patients). Beginning to practise a therapy of this kind can be rather like a religious conversion; and converts, as we know, are often more zealous in their advocacy of their new faith than are those who have grown up in it. People who have become enamoured of traditional acupuncture generally regard the attempt to modernize the ideas as a compromise too far.

There are others, however, who prefer not to abandon their science-based way of thinking and who wish to practise acupuncture, if possible, without giving up the modern understanding of how the body works. This is my own position, and the book is written for people who think in this way.

For traditionalists, the very antiquity of the ancient system is part of its appeal. After all, if a form of medicine has been in existence for thousands of years, it must be valuable, mustn't it? I'm not sure how valid this argument is, but, in any case, claims for the antiquity of acupuncture need to be qualified. Acupuncture as we have it today is largely mediaeval, though with elements that are older than this and also some that are more recent (nineteenth century). The oldest medical texts we have were discovered in the Mawangdui tombs as late as 1973 and were composed or copied at some time between the third century BCE and 168 BCE. Although these texts describe 'channels' (*mo*) that are clearly the forerunners of the 'channels' (*jingmo*) of acupuncture, the astonishing thing is that they say nothing at all about acupuncture 'points' or, indeed, about acupuncture; the treatment they describe is moxibustion. Acupuncture theory therefore appears to have evolved progressively and is unlikely to have originated much before the first century BCE (Kuriyama, 2000). But all this is largely beside the point; what matters is how we should regard the ideas on which it is based.

Here we need to separate observation from theory. Although traditional acupuncture is no doubt based on sound observation in many cases, the explanatory framework it depends on is no longer useful. As an analogy, compare the geocentric Ptolemaic theory of the solar system, which explained the planetary movements by means of an enormously complicated system of epicycles, interlocking with one another like gearwheels. This accounted for the known facts but at the cost of introducing a horrendous amount of unnecessary complexity. The Copernican system, with the sun at the centre and the planets and the earth revolving round it, works a great deal better. Traditional acupuncture theory, I suggest, is the equivalent in medicine of the Ptolemaic theory in astronomy. The ancient Chinese were acute observers and described accurately the acupuncture phenomena which we can see today, but their explanations were unnecessarily complicated, or complicated in the wrong way, being based on a set of assumptions about the world that are not part of modern science. The ancient theory can be made to work, after a fashion, but why bother when there is a more elegant and rational modern explanation available?

The traditional system is not only complicated in the wrong way, it is also static. This is perhaps an even greater drawback. As Ted Kaptchuk (Kaptchuk, 1983), one of the best Western writers on ancient Chinese medicine, has pointed out, everything in the traditional system comes back in the end to yin and yang. Nothing really new can be added; if an apparently new phenomenon is found or a new kind of treatment is invented, it has to be interpreted in terms of yin and yang. This is similar to the mediaeval European habit of referring all scientific knowledge to Aristotle and all medical knowledge to Galen; if it wasn't described by these authorities it isn't true. Such an attitude is a recipe for stagnation. Science, in contrast, proceeds by challenging authority. We don't have better brains than the ancients, we don't have more subtle moral intuitions, we are not better artists, but we do know incomparably more about the natural world, and it's simply perverse to put all that knowledge aside and imprison oneself in a prescientific world view.

In saying this, I have no wish to trivialize or to denigrate the ancient Chinese world view. That would be an absurdly arrogant position to adopt. But we need to distinguish between philosophy and science. Philosophical ideas don't go out of date in the way that scientific theories do. We can study the thought of Plato and Aristotle with profit, even though they lived so long ago, and the same is true of ancient Chinese thought. Aristotle's science, on the other hand, is of historical interest only. The Chinese conception of the body, and of health and disease, satisfied a substantial part of the world's population for many centuries, and we can certainly profit from studying them and comparing them with our own. But the attempt to practise traditional acupuncture in the West, in the twenty-first century, seems to me to be misguided.

There are several reasons for this. One is the sheer difficulty, for a modern Westerner, of accommodating oneself to this way of thinking. Not only is it alien, but the medium through which we receive it is questionable. Almost all Westerners will, inevitably, have to rely on translations, and there is no guarantee that the ancient ideas can survive this process unscathed; indeed, some are practically untranslatable. Much of the terminology and many of the concepts used by Western acupuncture enthusiasts derive from the writings of a French diplomat, Soulié de Morant, and these contain a number of important mistranslations and misconceptions. But even if we ignore this, it is deceptively easy to fall into the illusion that traditional Chinese medicine and acupuncture form a monolithic body of 'holistic' truth standing in opposition to Western 'reductionism'. The facts are otherwise. Acupuncture is much more complex and varied than many Western enthusiasts suppose. For one thing, different versions, with different practices and philosophies, developed in a number of Far Eastern countries (Japan, Korea, Vietnam). For another, even within China, acupuncture underwent many transformations during its long history, nor was it always accorded the respect it receives today; at one time it was even banned by law. And, in any case, very little is still known in the West about Chinese medicine: there are said to be over 1200 texts on the subject, of which only about 200 have ever been translated.

These are important considerations, but there is another that seems to me even more important. To put it quite simply, the ancient Chinese physicians ignored anatomy as we understand the term. Modern Chinese books on acupuncture, written for a Western audience, do contain illustrations of the body that are quite similar to those that might appear in a Western medical textbook, apart from the lines indicating the 'meridians', but this is a very recent development, reflecting the progressive westernization of modern Chinese medicine. Older books provided very different illustrations. Typically, they depicted an almost comically corpulent individual, clad in a loincloth, over whose rather shapeless frame meandered the lines of the so-called meridians. The startling omission, to a Western medical reader, is the lack of any indication of the real structure of the body: no bones, no muscles, no internal organs. The drawings, in fact, are not anatomical.

The reason for this is quite simple. According to Kuriyama (2000), the ancient Chinese hardly practised dissection at all and, in almost the sole account of it that we do have, the focus of interest is not on anatomy in the modern sense of the word. What the dissectors were interested in was the precise dimensions and capacities of the various organs; probably, Kuriyama suggests, because they hoped that these dimensions would give a clue to the unknowable dimensions of the universe, which the microcosm of the body was supposed to reflect. In any case, this experiment was seldom or never repeated. Until the twentieth century Chinese physicians didn't recognize the existence of muscles. This may appear astonishing, until we remember that other major medical traditions (Ayurvedic, Egyptian) also managed without anatomy for thousands of years. Seen in this context, it is the arising of anatomical study in the West that needs explanation rather than its absence in China.

In the West, anatomical study was part of the great scientific revolution that began in the sixteenth century and has continued to accelerate ever since. We are the heirs to the inquisitive observers of the Renaissance who wished, above all, to probe and discover Nature's secrets. Some, it's true, question the status of science today, and claim that scientific knowledge is as culture-determined as any other body of opinion. This seems to me to be nonsense. Science is also under attack on other grounds, and certainly it is true that scientific discoveries are potentially dangerous and their results unpredictable; we may in the end turn out to be the cat whom curiosity killed. But it's too late to turn back now. Knowledge once gained cannot be un-known. We know the muscles are there, and it is impossible, even for traditionalists, to practise acupuncture without recognizing this fact.

References

James R. (1998) There is more to acupuncture than the weekend course. *Complementary Therapies in Medicine*, 6; 203–7.

Kaptchuk T.J. (1983) *Chinese Medicine: the web that has no weaver*. Hutchinson Publishing Group, London.

Kuriyama S. (2000) *The Expressiveness of the Body and the Divergence of Greek and Chinese Medicine*. Zone Books, New York.

Chapter 2

An outline of the traditional system

Although, for the reasons explained in Chapter 1, this book is on the modern version of acupuncture, it is essential to include a short account of the traditional system, for several reasons, quite apart from any feeling that we ought to make a polite bow (or kowtow) to the originators of the treatment. One is that it is impossible to be 'literate' in acupuncture without at least a nodding acquaintance with the ancient ideas. Another is that much of what is written about acupuncture assumes a basic knowledge of the terminology, and even writers and lecturers who don't adhere to the traditional version may still use this terminology to a certain extent. If you know nothing at all about the ancient system you will feel lost and 'out of it' as you read or listen. Still another, and more practical, reason for having a nodding familiarity with the terminology is that it provides a convenient form of shorthand. To anyone familiar with that terminology, the statement that a needle was placed in Gall Bladder 21 conveys an instant piece of knowledge; to say that the needle was placed in the midpoint of the trapezius muscle would be more cumbersome. Similarly, to say that de qi was obtained would immediately tell an acupuncturist that certain sensations were produced in the patient and felt by the operator, and would also imply that certain consequences might be expected to follow; there is simply no Western equivalent for this expression.

Our knowledge of the ancient system is still evolving. Until the discovery of the Mawangdui tomb texts alluded to in Chapter 1, the earliest source for ancient Chinese medical theory was the *Yellow Emperor's Classic of Internal Medicine* – the *Neijing*. This was assembled from a variety of texts from different medical traditions and was probably first compiled during the Han dynasty (221 BCE–220 CE). However, the original text no longer survives and the organization and some of the contents of the present *Neijing* are the product of later recensions. Another early text, the *Nanjing*, was an attempt to elucidate the *Neijing* (*nan* = difficulties). Subsequently, other writers continued to comment on the *Neijing* to bring out and clarify its ideas and sometimes to add new ones. This process has been compared by Ted Kaptchuk (1983) to the way the Bible has been treated in rabbinical exegesis or by the Church Fathers.

Without such commentaries the *Neijing* would be almost incomprehensible to modern readers. Modern textbooks are based in part on works written in the Ching (Manchu) period (1644–1911). But even this material is largely inaccessible to modern Chinese, who, since the orthographic reforms of the Cultural Revolution, are unable to read the older texts with any facility.

For Westerners, an additional complication, as I mentioned in Chapter 1, derives from translation. For all these reasons, a description of traditional acupuncture as practised in the West is necessarily over-simplified in a number of ways; some have referred to this version of acupuncture, disparagingly, as Europuncture.

In this chapter I present an overview of the traditional system as Westerners will generally encounter it. This is deliberately very schematic, and a good deal is omitted; I make no attempt, for example, to dive into the complexities of the five phases. I do, however, include a few notes on ideas that are generally not included in presentations for students but which I think help to place the subject in a truer perspective.

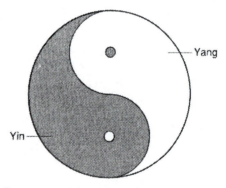

Yin–yang symbol

The basic concepts

Qi

The fundamental idea of traditional Chinese acupuncture, and indeed of most ancient Chinese philosophy, is the concept of qi or chi. The term is impossible to translate. It has something in common with the Indian idea of *prana* and the ancient Greek idea of *pneuma*. All things in the world, including the human body, are said to be composed of qi. Qi is always flowing and changing, and it is what animates living beings. Qi could be thought of as lying at the border between matter and energy, but it is impossible to define the concept clearly, partly because classical Chinese thought doesn't seem to go in for definitions much. The ancient Chinese preferred to describe things in terms of what they do rather than what they are. Thus, qi sustains all kinds of movement and change, it protects against harmful influences, it transforms food into other substances as well as into qi itself, it holds organs in place and prevents excessive fluid loss, and it warms the body. It flows with the blood in the blood vessels and also in special channels (meridians) called *jing*. (Qi is yang, blood is yin.) A fascinating feature of this scheme is that qi and blood were thought of as circulating in a pumped system; thus the ancient Chinese are said to have anticipated William Harvey's discovery of the circulation of the blood by hundreds of years (indeed, as early as the second century BCE). However, this idea was arrived at on theoretical grounds, not as the result of experiments like those of Harvey.

Both excess and deficiency of qi are held to be harmful, and either condition can cause disease.

Yin–yang polarity

The concept of yin and yang is, like the theory of qi, of fundamental importance in ancient Chinese philosophy; yin and yang are supposed to operate throughout the whole universe, not just in the human body. Originally yang meant the sunny side of a slope or the north bank of a river, while yin meant the shady side of a slope or the south bank of a river. These meanings were later extended to cover a vast range of polarities, so that, for example, yang came to refer to heat, movement, vigour, increase and upward or outward movement, while yin referred to cold, rest, passivity, decrease, and inward and downward movement. On the biological level yang is male, yin female.

Although yin and yang are polar opposites they are not mutually exclusive. Yin always contains at least a trace of yang and vice versa. In the traditional yin–yang diagram this is indicated by the fact that yang contains a small spot of yin and yin a small spot of yang.

Perhaps the nearest Western equivalents would be the concepts of positive and negative in electricity and north and south in magnetism; negative implies positive and you cannot isolate one pole of a magnet. But yin and yang are not thought of as static fixed entities; they constantly interact with each other and transform themselves into each other. In the whole of nature, as well as in ourselves, there is an ever-changing flow of yang into yin and yin into yang.

Modern accounts of the traditional system written for Westerners usually state that our state of health depends on the balance between yin and yang. If either preponderates more than it should the result may be disease, which is thus thought of as resulting from a dynamic imbalance. (Underactivity or overactivity of endocrine glands, such as the thyroid, might be a modern instance of this principle.) Treatment is conceived of as a means of restoring the balance. While this description is true so far as it goes, it is a considerable simplification and largely neglects the effects of 'wind', discussed below.

The organs

Traditional Chinese medicine names many of the organs familiar to us, but we have to be careful about applying the modern concept of 'organ' in the traditional context. As we saw in Chapter 1, the ancient Chinese didn't practise anatomical dissection to any extent, and the modern notion of a well-defined structure can't be equated exactly with the Chinese view, which is concerned, not with what the viscera are, but with what they do in health and sickness. The Chinese terms are *zang* and *fu*; the *zang* include liver, heart, spleen, lungs, and kidneys and the *fu* include gall bladder, small intestine, stomach, large intestine, and urinary bladder. The difference between the two groups is that the *zang* are solid and the *fu* are hollow. Discussion of these in the *Neijing* has less to do with discrete structures seen in dissection than with their supposed functions. Thus, 'gall bladder disease' could as easily refer to dizziness or ringing in the ears as to the gall bladder itself.

So far we have encountered only ten 'organs', but there was also an eleventh: *sanjiao*, the controversial viscus 'with a name but no form', usually referred to as the triple energizer or triple warmer in Western texts and there located approximately in the centre of the body. And finally, just to round the number up to twelve, modern acupuncture texts include the pericardium as the sixth *zang*.

The channels (meridians)

The term 'meridian', though widely used, is completely misleading; 'channel' is a better translation of the Chinese term (*jing*), since the idea is that there are subtle vessels running throughout the body to connect the organs and carry qi. Once again, however, we have to keep in mind the Chinese relative lack of interest in structure, and recognize that what they are talking about is not so much a system of vessels as a system of flowing currents. In other words, it's the flow that is important, not the conduit in which it occurs.

The points (xue)

Once more we encounter difficulties with translation. The Chinese term *xue* means holes or caverns, and this connects with the idea of wind (to be discussed shortly); the *xue* are sites at which winds stream in and out of strategic orifices in the skin. The English 'point' suggests something different and has occasioned much misunderstanding.

Diagrams of the channels represent them as if they were lying on the surface of the body, but in fact they are to be thought of as running at a

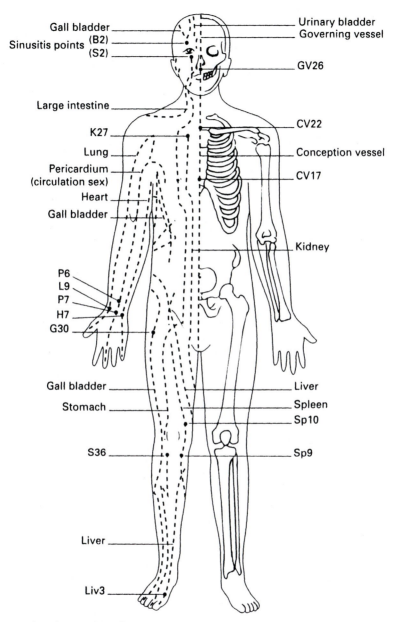

Gall bladder

Sinusitis points (B2) (S2)

Large intestine

K27

Lung

Pericardium (circulation sex)

Heart

Gall bladder

P6
L9
P7
H7
G30

Gall bladder

Stomach

S36

Liver

Liv3

Urinary bladder

Governing vessel

GV26

CV22

Conception vessel

CV17

Kidney

Liver

Spleen

Sp10

Sp9

The main channels – front view

variable depth inside the body and only coming to the surface at certain places. (They have been compared to the District Line of London's underground system.) The 'points' mostly lie on the channels at places where they run near the surface. A few points (the so-called extrameridian points) do not lie on channels. Some 365 acupuncture points are

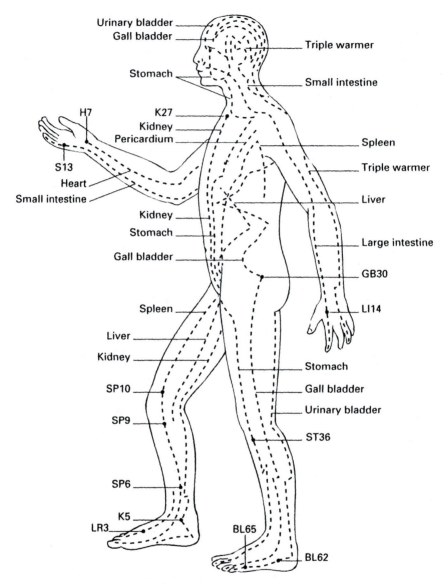

The main channels – side view

described, but in practice many fewer are used. (The correspondence with the number of days in the year is doubtless not coincidental.) The points all have Chinese names which often sound poetic in translation (Sea of Blood, Gate of Dumbness, Crooked Spring), but Western acupuncture books use a more prosaic system of numbering, which is more or less standardized.

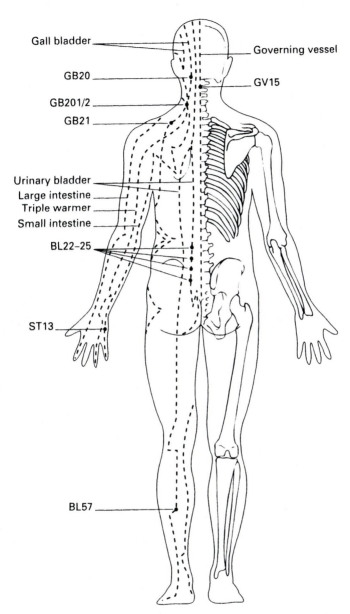

Gall bladder

Governing vessel

GB20

GV15

GB201/2

GB21

Urinary bladder
Large intestine
Triple warmer
Small intestine

BL22–25

ST13

BL57

The main channels – back view

Location of the channels

A total of 59 acupuncture channels is described; of these only 14 possess acupuncture points. Of the 14, 12 are paired and 2 are midline, therefore unpaired. Their names are given in Table 2.1.

Table 2.1. *Acupuncture channels*

Paired	Lung LU (Lu, P)
	Large Intestine LI (CO, Co, IC)
	Stomach ST (S, St, E, M)
	Spleen SP (Sp, LP)
	Heart HT (H, C, Ht, HE)
	Small Intestine SI (Si, IT)
	Urinary Bladder BL (B, Bl, UB)
	Kidney KI (K, Ki, Rn)
	Pericardium PC (P, PE, HC)
	Triple Energizer TE (T, TW, SJ, 3H, TB)
	Liver LR (Liv, LV, H)
	Gall Bladder GB (G, GB, VF)
Unpaired	Governing Vessel GV (Du, Du Go, Gv, TM)
	Conception Vessel CV (Co, Cv, J, REN, Ren)

The abbreviations given in Table 2.1 are those in common use. There is now a WHO list of abbreviations but it is not used universally. The sequence used in the table is that found in books on traditional Chinese medicine because it corresponds to the way that qi is supposed to flow. However, the overall picture is easier to grasp if we ignore the traditional description and instead think of the channels as if they were real anatomical structures that might be described in a modern textbook. If we do this, we find that they can be arranged in two main classes: an upper limb group and a lower limb group. The upper limb group can be further subdivided into an anterior and a posterior group, but this is more difficult in the lower limb group. Table 2.2 sets out this arrangement and also indicates the main areas in which the various channels run, together with the sequence of point numbering (distal–proximal or vice versa).

Certain features of Table 2.2 should be noted. Some of the lower limb channels (GB, ST, and BL) have a very long course and wide distribution, literally from head to foot. Certain channels cross each other, especially LR and SP. GB is the only truly lateral channel, BL the only truly posterior channel. For much of its course on the back, BL is doubled.

The five phases theory

This is complementary to the yin–yang idea. The five phases interact with one another according to a complex scheme. Their names are Wood, Fire, Earth, Metal and Water, and they are related to the various organs and to one another. The interplay of the phases has implications for treatment in the traditional system. The theory usually attracts a lot of attention in Western books on the traditional system, perhaps because it is complicated and allows plenty of opportunity for mystification. Modern

Table 2.2. *Areas through which the two main channels of the upper and lower limb groups run*

	Channel	Site	Distribution	Sequence
Upper limbs: anterior group	LU	radial	shoulder/hand	prox–dist
	PC	median	shoulder/hand	prox–dist
	HT	ulnar	axilla/hand	prox–dist
Upper limbs: posterior group	LI	radial	hand/face	dist–prox
	TE	median	hand/face	dist–prox
	SI	ulnar	hand/face	dist–prox
Lower limbs: long group	GB	lateral	head/foot	prox–dist
	ST	anterior	head/foot	prox–dist
	BL	posterior	head/foot	prox–dist
Lower limbs: short group	KI	medial	foot/chest	dist–prox
	LR	medial	foot/chest	dist–proxv
	SP	medial	foot/chest	dist–prox
Midline	CV	anterior	perineum/chin	inf–sup
	GV	posterior	coccyx/upper lip	inf–sup

Chinese books, at least in Western languages, usually say little or nothing about it. 'The European adoption of this method stems partly from a desire for an exotic scheme and partly from lack of adequate information' (Kaptchuk, 1983).

Disease causation: wind

There are usually said to be three classes of disease causation: environment, emotions, and way of life. The environmental influences are wind, cold, heat, and dampness; way of life includes diet, physical activity, and sexual activity. Descriptions based on these concepts suggest a 'holistic' view of disease, albeit one that is difficult to relate to modern ideas of pathology, but in any case this scheme is a later construct. The prime cause of disease in the traditional system is wind. In the *Neijing* it is identified as 'the beginning of the hundred diseases'.

The importance of wind in classical Chinese medicine can hardly be exaggerated. Western commentators on Chinese medicine, Kuriyama believes, tend to play down the importance of wind in the classical scheme, preferring to concentrate on yin and yang and the five phases; but, although these are certainly essential components of the classical system, the influence of wind is crucial (Kuriyama, 2000). Wind in this context is much more than an atmospheric phenomenon. It is thought of as a cosmic influence that is capable of inducing chaos, disrupting the

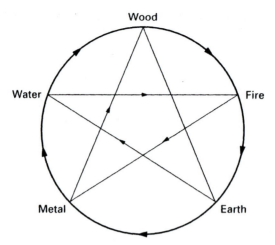

The five phases

orderly function of society and also of the internal economy of the individual, by exciting imbalances. Thus, it isn't so much a cause of disease as disease itself, an alien invader, which enters the body by the pores and by the *xue* (acupuncture points). Part of the reason for doing acupuncture is to empty the noxious wind that has invaded from without.

Methods of diagnosis

The traditional Chinese physician, like his Western counterpart, takes a history and notes the patient's general appearance and demeanour. The colour of the face was held to be of great importance in ancient times; a skilful physician was supposed to be able to diagnose illness and predict its course by looking at the patient's face. Particular attention is also paid to the tongue: its colour, coating and so on. The most important examination, however, is that of the pulse.

This is felt at the wrist at three locations on each side and both superficially and deeply, giving a total of 12 pulses which are related to the 12 internal organs. (Some sources give even larger numbers of pulses.) The quality of the pulse is described in terms such as slippery, rough, and wiry. A skilful physician is said to be able to derive an astonishing amount of information from the pulse alone, but learning the art requires thorough training, long experience, and the gift of intuition or sensitivity. The information it provides is of course couched in terms of traditional diagnoses, and it is difficult or impossible to translate these into modern concepts.

Treatment according to the traditional system

On the basis of these examinations the physician decides which organs are out of balance. Needles are then inserted to 'stimulate' or 'sedate' the relevant organs by adjusting the flow of qi. This is essentially a hydraulic concept; the acupuncturist is thought of as a kind of engineer, opening and closing the valves as appropriate. (There is, of course, nothing mystical about this. People who are attracted to traditional acupuncture because they think it is in some way mystical are under a considerable misapprehension.)

In most cases today a number of needles are inserted and left in for 20 minutes or so. (Certain ancient texts say that a really expert practitioner needs to insert only one needle.) Much emphasis is laid on the accurate placement of the needles. The location of the acupuncture points is specified in terms of the *cun*, or 'Chinese inch', which is a variable measurement based on the dimensions of the particular patient. For example, the distance between the intermediate and distal skin folds in the middle index finger constitutes one *cun*, and so does the width of the thumb at the interphalangeal joint. Nowadays Chinese textbooks tend to use detailed anatomical atlases like those found in Western books.

A great deal of attention is paid to obtaining various types of sensations from the patient as the needles are inserted, and the physician also experiences various sensations as he manipulates the needle. These phenomena, which are collectively called de qi, are supposed to be due to tapping into the flow of qi. Four typical sensations are described, and their names have been translated as numbness, fullness, heaviness and sourness (a kind of muscular ache like that caused by over-exertion).

The time at which treatment was applied was considered to be important in the traditional system. Indeed, the Chinese remarkably anticipated another modern discovery here: circadian rhythms. Observations of cycles in disease intensity are recorded in the *Neijing*.

Moxibustion

Moxibustion is similar to acupuncture; as noted in Chapter 1, it may be older than acupuncture. Material obtained from certain plants (*Artemisia* spp.) is ignited and used to warm the tissues. It may be placed directly on the skin or on layers of various substances (salt, garlic), or may be wrapped round the handle of the needle. Sometimes this is done at ordinary acupuncture points but there are also some special moxibustion points.

Traditional acupuncture in the light of modern knowledge

In this chapter and the preceding I have attempted to provide a brief outline of a vast and ancient system of thought. Inevitably this has to be impressionistic, but I hope that I have at least succeeded in showing that traditional Chinese medicine is difficult or impossible to correlate with modern ways of thinking about the body. This, however, has not prevented a number of people from trying. Numerous attempts to verify the objective existence of acupuncture points and channels have been made in both East and West, but it seems to me that this enterprise is fundamentally mistaken, since the ancient Chinese outlook was so different from our own that correlations of this kind cannot be made. At any rate, the attempts have mostly ended in failure. Early claims that the points and channels could be demonstrated histologically have not stood up to later verification. Electrical studies intended to detect the points have given variable results. At present, the most that can be said is that there may be some electrical changes at certain acupuncture points but the significance of this is unknown.

Many of the classic points correspond to what are known in the Western literature as trigger points – a subject I return to in more detail in subsequent chapters – and some modern acupuncturists go so far as to equate acupuncture points with trigger points. The problem with this idea, however, is that trigger points are tender areas in muscles, whereas, as we have seen, the ancient Chinese didn't recognize the existence of muscles.

Yet another possibility is that the acupuncture channels represent projection patterns within the central nervous system. There is some evidence that patients suffering from arthritis indicate, more often than not, that their pain distribution matches the classic acupuncture channels, at least to some extent. In the past I was inclined to believe that this may have been the way in which the channel idea arose, but I now find it less likely; Kuriyama's suggestion (Kuriyama, 2000) that they developed (at least partly) out of bloodletting appears to me more plausible. The idea of the *mo* (the vessels that are the forerunners of the *jing* (the channels of acupuncture) was originally intertwined with that of the blood vessels visible at the surface of the body. Many of the most important needling points lie on surface veins and arteries, and the texts sometimes described the same sites as useful for both acupuncture and bloodletting.

Pulse diagnosis, likewise, is difficult or impossible to verify in a modern context. Our modern classification of disease is based on anatomy and pathology. There is no way of relating such a diagnosis to that of the traditional categories of ancient Chinese medicine; the two are simply incommensurate.

As we saw in Chapter 1, modern Chinese texts on acupuncture, at least those meant for Westerners, have departed from the traditional way of presenting the subject in a number of ways; they generally say little or nothing about pulse diagnosis or the five phases and they include illustrations that are fairly similar to those in Western anatomical books. This modernization is symptomatic of a partial abandonment of the ancient system. According to Nathan Sivin, an American sinologist who has studied the question at first hand, modern Chinese doctors do not use or understand the ancient system (Sivin, 1990). They are unable to read the classical literature, which has to be translated into modern Chinese. Although acupuncture is still used, the diagnostic methods are modern. Patients likewise are no longer familiar with the yin–yang and five phases concepts. Sivin, himself an enthusiast for the traditional system, concludes regretfully that there can be no return to this system in its original form.

References

Kaptchuk T.J. (1983) *Chinese Medicine: the web that has no weaver.* Hutchinson Publishing Group, London.

Kuriyama S. (2000) *The Expressiveness of the Body and the Divergence of Greek and Chinese Medicine.* Zone Books, New York.

Sivin N. (1990) *American Journal of Acupuncture,* 18; 325–41.

Chapter 3

Modern acupuncture

We turn now to medical acupuncture or modern acupuncture. These terms are preferable to 'Western acupuncture', because the treatment in question is based on the modern understanding of anatomy, physiology, and pathology – that is, on science; and science is neither Western nor Eastern, but just science.

In this version of acupuncture we can largely forget about the traditional apparatus of yin and yang, channels ('meridians'), and 'points'. Even if these are not ignored completely, they are reinterpreted in radically different ways. Another, very important, difference is that the modern version does not use any special diagnostic methods such as the pulse or the appearance of the tongue. Modern acupuncture uses conventional diagnostic methods. Still another difference concerns the needling process itself: the ancient system had the concepts of sedation and stimulation, but these are ignored in the modern version.

The foregoing differences are largely negative, but modern acupuncture also has positive aspects; it includes theories about how inserting needles into a patient may relieve symptoms. It is possible to put forward a reasonably plausible explanation for this, at least in relation to pain; effects on other symptoms are harder to account for. It hardly needs saying, I suppose, that we are not yet in a position to explain all the phenomena that are seen by acupuncturists. For example, patients very frequently report radiation of sensations from the site of needling that don't correspond to any nerve distribution or to the spinal segment in which the needling was done. Such observations must indicate the existence of patterns of activation within the central nervous system whose nature is still unknown, but which must exist to explain the reported sensations. Explanations of these effects must await future discoveries about the organization of the nervous system.

I have stated the differences between modern and traditional acupuncture pretty starkly, but the distinction between the two versions is sometimes less sharp than this implies. In fact, what we find in acupuncture is more like a spectrum of opinion. At one extreme there are adherents of the traditional system in its fullest form; most of these, although not all, are people who have approached acupuncture without first undergoing a conventional training as a health professional. At the other end of the spectrum are those who reject the traditional system outright and who have often devised their own terminology; for example, some prefer to speak of 'dry needling' rather than acupuncture. In between there are many who accept some parts of the traditional system but not others. My own position, as will become clear as we go on, is fairly far towards the 'modern' end of the spectrum although not quite at its furthest limit.

What I suppose is that the ancient Chinese stumbled, perhaps in part through the practice of bloodletting, on the fact that puncturing the skin at certain sites could alleviate symptoms of disease. They explained this in terms of their existing world view, and hence there gradually developed, over many centuries, the set of teachings that we now call acupuncture.

Modern acupuncture is now beginning to emerge from this ancient collection of ideas. It has a long way to go before it is widely accepted, but I believe the time will come when modern acupuncture will be seen to bear much the same relation to the traditional system as chemistry bears to alchemy or astrology to astronomy. (This doesn't mean, of course, that traditional acupuncture will wither away overnight; astrology, after all, is still very much with us.)

This view will certainly be criticised by enthusiasts for the traditional system on the grounds that it oversimplifies acupuncture almost to the point of caricature. My reply is that there is very little objective evidence for the efficacy of any form of acupuncture, traditional or modern, and even less to show that one way of needling is better than another. Indeed, such evidence as does exist mostly shows no differences according to whether the needles are inserted at 'correct' acupuncture points or elsewhere. We are therefore still obliged to rely on personal experience in this matter, and mine suggests that the non-traditional version is at least as effective as the traditional.

Critics of acupuncture naturally take an entirely different view, and dismiss the whole of acupuncture as primitive superstition. For such ultra-sceptics, all acupuncture is nonsensical; its apparent successes can be confidently ascribed to the 'placebo effect' and spontaneous recovery. These days we are all supposed to adhere to the standards of 'evidence-based medicine', and it is difficult to refute the accusation that acupuncture (along with most other forms of unconventional medicine) has relatively little in the way of evidence to support it. Much of what is claimed by acupuncturists of all types is still 'anecdotal' – a pejorative term in the present climate.

I have to admit to a certain amount of sympathy with this view. If I knew nothing about the subject, I, too, might be tempted to dismiss it as nonsensical. The fact that it does seem to work in practice is surprising. However, as I mentioned previously, it is now possible to put forward a reasonable explanation of how stimulating the nervous system via needles might have therapeutic effects.

Theories of mechanism of action

If acupuncture does work, what can we say about the possible mechanisms of action? The great majority of modern theorizing about acupuncture has concentrated on its ability to relieve pain. Many modern acupuncturists appear rather unhappy about claims that acupuncture can be used to treat disorders not characterized by pain, such as allergies or bronchial asthma; it is as if the conceptual leap required to envisage such possibilities was too great for them to take. Nevertheless, as we shall see in Part 3, acupuncture does seem to work for a number of these non-painful disorders. However, there is very little theorizing to explain how it could conceivably work in such cases, whereas there is quite a lot of fairly well-founded explanation in the case of pain. I therefore concentrate on pain in what follows.

Changing views of the mechanism of pain perception
(Devor, 1995; Wall & Melzack, 1984; Wall, 2000)

Older models of pain perception, which go back as far as René Descartes for their inspiration, were essentially simple input–output constructions. In one celebrated example, pain perception is portrayed as analogous to ringing a church bell to sound an alarm; a tug on the rope (the nerve) operates the bell (an area in the brain). Rather more sophisticated versions of this, in which the rope and bell are replaced by a telephone exchange, appeared in the twentieth century, but all such models have a common weakness: who is listening at the other end? Theories of this kind almost inevitably lead to the picture of a little man (homunculus) sitting inside the brain and registering the arrival of a pain impulse and saying 'Ouch!'

At the neurological level, what is supposed to happen is something like the following. You tread on a drawing pin, say. Pain impulses then travel via sensory nerves to the spinal cord, where they relay with nerve tracts that take them upwards, perhaps to the thalamus. Here further relays take them to the cerebral cortex, where they are consciously registered as pain. After further processing, impulses will then travel down the motor system to the muscles to make you withdraw your foot (and possibly travel to your vocal apparatus to make you swear).

Quite apart from any problems with the homunculus, this simple input–output model doesn't accord with the known facts. For example, it doesn't explain how injuries received in battle or in sport sometimes cause no pain at all at the time, nor does it account for the suppression of pain by hypnosis. It also fails to explain why many patients complain bitterly of pain long after the injury that originally gave rise to the pain has healed. In the past, such patients were often dismissed as malingerers or hypochondriacs, but today there is ample theory to explain why they continue to experience pain.

There is another illogicality at work here as well. If we say that pain persisting for long after an injury has healed is 'all in the mind', we are really postulating a kind of ghost in the machine. We are implying that there is some kind of ethereal spirit floating above the body and brain that somehow introduces a false perception of pain into the system. Such dualistic thinking is very unpopular today in science and in modern psychology, so it is odd that many doctors still speak as if it were valid in the context of pain.

In the nineteenth century the anatomist Hughlings Jackson advanced the idea that the nervous system is built as a hierarchy. At the lowest level we have the spinal cord; above this there is the brain stem, then the central parts of the brain (hypothalamus and thalamus), and finally the resplendent cortex, the proudest acquisition of humans, sitting atop it all and acting as the ultimate authority. Today, in contrast, we tend to think of the nervous system as more like a commonwealth, in which all the component parts interact but in which there is no dominant level. In part, probably, this is a political as well as a scientific change in outlook: it reflects a modern tendency towards egalitarianism and anti-elitism, but it is probably also a truer reflection of how the nervous system actually works. In relation to pain perception, it implies that whether pain is experienced at any given moment is the outcome of a complex interplay of activity at many different levels in the nervous system.

A new way of thinking about pain
(Wall & Melzack, 1984; Wall, 2000)

A different way of thinking about pain has emerged in recent decades: one that affords more useful ways of trying to explain acupuncture. The starting point here was the work of P.D. Wall and R. Melzack. They put forward what they called the gate theory of pain, which was destined to become very influential. In outline, this postulated the existence of gates or filters in the posterior horns of the spinal cord. When these were open, pain information could be transmitted upwards to the brain; when they were closed, transmission was blocked. The gates were supposed to be controlled by incoming messages from the periphery. In the simplest possible terms, the gates were supposed to be closed by impulses coming from large-diameter fibres and opened by small-diameter fibres. We could picture the large-diameter fibres as acting like a brake and the small-diameter fibres as acting like an accelerator. The theory was the basis for the technique of transcutaneous electrical nerve stimulation (TENS) for the relief of pain. The theory has been modified and expanded in various ways but its essential features are still widely accepted today.

In a little more detail, the system works like this. There are sensory neurons in the posterior horns of the spinal cord whose axons travel upwards towards the brain. These are called SG (substantia gelatinosa) cells because they are found in a layer of the posterior horn that has that name, and they are responsible for the transmission upwards of information about tissue damage. The activity of these neurons is modified by smaller excitatory and inhibitory neurons. When there is tissue damage, news of this reaches the spinal cord via C (unmyelinated) and A-delta (small myelinated) fibres. These activate the SG neurons in the posterior horns, but whether or not these neurons transmit information onwards depends on the balance of the input from the small inhibitory and excitatory cells. These, in turn, are influenced by the large-diameter and small-diameter fibres, but it is not only information coming in from the periphery that influence the gates; so, too, do descending impulses from higher up in the central nervous system. This is very important for hypotheses about acupuncture analgesia.

Pain pathways and mechanisms in relation to acupuncture
(Bowsher, 1998; Ernst & White, 1999)

In thinking about pain, we have to distinguish between nociception (perception of tissue damage) and pain; the two don't necessarily go hand in hand. Thus, tissue damage doesn't always cause pain, and pain can persist in the absence of tissue damage. We also have to distinguish between the experience of pain and the emotional accompaniment of pain: it is possible to feel pain without being particularly distressed by it. So the links between injury and pain, and between pain and suffering, are a good deal more complicated than is often realized.

Three types of nerve fibre are involved in nociception. A-beta fibres are large-diameter myelinated fibres. A-delta fibres are also myelinated but are smaller in diameter. C fibres are unmyelinated small-diameter fibres. Both A-delta and C fibre systems are concerned with nociception and pain perception but they have different roles. The A-delta fibre system is responsible for accurate localization of noxious stimulation without much emotional accompaniment, whereas the C fibre system yields poorly localized perception of pain accompanied with stronger emotional effects. The difference between the two systems can be appreciated when you injure yourself, for example, by stubbing your toe. There is an initial burst of acute pain, followed after a few seconds by a more diffuse pain which has a 'deep' quality and is considerably more unpleasant than the first pain. The rapid-onset pain is mediated by the A-delta system, the second pain by the C fibre system.

A-delta fibres are activated by heavy pressure, heat and cold, and also by pinprick, which is where acupuncture comes in. A-delta fibres are thought to be responsible for acupuncture analgesia; the A-beta fibres are probably involved only in TENS and electro-acupuncture analgesia and not in ordinary clinical acupuncture. Pinprick, of course, is painful, and it may appear paradoxical that this system should also be thought to be involved in acupuncture analgesia, but the explanation is that the A-delta system has an inhibitory feedback effect on the pain transmission mechanism. A-delta activity goes to part of the hypothalamus (the arcuate nucleus), which in turn activates descending impulses that switch on inhibitory systems in the brain stem.

There are probably several of these brain-stem systems but two are well known. One is mediated by serotonin and involves midline bodies of neurons including the periaqueductal grey and the nucleus raphe magnus; the other is mediated by noradrenaline and descends on either side of the midline, through the gigantocellular and paragigantocellular nuclei; the locus coeruleus in the pons is also part of this system.

Both these systems ultimately act on the SG cells in the posterior horns of the spinal cord. Thus, we have a complete control loop, in which the A-delta pathway ends in the hypothalamus and activates the descending inhibitory pathways. The nucleus raphe magnus, one of the way stations on the serotonin pathway, is organized somatotopically (that is, it contains a map of the body), and this may explain the strong analgesic effects of certain acupuncture points.

Many of the areas just mentioned (arcuate nucleus of the hypothalamus, periaqueductal grey, and nucleus raphe magnus) have reciprocal projections with other brain areas such as the prefrontal cortex, the hypothalamus, the septum, and the limbic system; these connections provide a basis for understanding how the perception of pain can be influenced by emotion, attention, expectation, and memory. Acupuncture can be thought of as yet another means of activating these descending inhibitory systems.

Whether particular needling sites in the body are more effective than others in inducing analgesia is still uncertain. Experiments have shown that a noxious stimulus anywhere in the body can produce analgesia. This phenomenon is called diffuse noxious inhibitory control (DNIC). It is mediated by opioids and is thought to involve an area in the caudal medulla called the subnucleus reticularis dorsalis, which projects downwards to the spinal cord at all levels. In relation to acupuncture, it has the consequence that almost any kind of needle stimulus may be expected to produce a certain amount of pain relief, whether or not it is done at a recognized acupuncture point. DNIC is a major reason why acupuncture research is difficult. However, the relevance to clinical practice is not great, since it appears that DNIC does not produce lasting pain relief after the stimulation ceases.

Much of the acupuncture research that has been done has been on short-term analgesia, especially in animals, and usually describes the result of treatment carried out on only one occasion. It has also often used fast electroacupuncture. This is considerably different from what happens in everyday clinical practice, when manual acupuncture is often used and is repeated on a number of occasions. It is this long-term effect of acupuncture which is particularly difficult to explain.

Various mechanisms have been suggested to explain the persistence of pain relief in clinical practice. For example, there could be long-term depression of the superficial spinal horn by low-frequency stimulation of afferent A fibres and induction of messenger RNA for opioid peptide expression. Increased serotonin levels in mast cells and platelets have been reported to occur after acupuncture.

The limbic system (Campbell, 1999)

Han (1987) proposed the idea of a 'mesolimbic loop' involving a number of structures including the amygdala, the periaqueductal grey and the nucleus raphe magnus. A reverberating circuit in this loop could maintain activity in the descending inhibitory system in the spinal cord for long periods. Even if this suggestion is wrong, the limbic system could be relevant to acupuncture in other ways.

The term 'limbic system' refers to a group of structures in the centre of the brain: cingulate gyrus, hippocampus, amygdala, and parts of the thalamus and hypothalamus. It was formerly thought to be the main brain site concerned with emotion, but now it is regarded chiefly as responsible for the formation of memory. However, it has some connection with emotion, especially in relation to the amygdala.

The limbic system is connected with all parts of the brain, including the cerebral cortex but also those areas in the brain stem that are responsible for modulation of pain perception. It therefore seems probable that the limbic system is implicated in acupuncture analgesia. It may be involved in certain other acupuncture phenomena as well.

As we shall see in subsequent chapters, patients receiving acupuncture may respond in quite surprising ways. They may experience relaxation or euphoria. They may cry or laugh for varying periods. They may, very exceptionally, have an epileptic fit. All these things are effects that can be produced by stimulating parts of the limbic system, especially the cingulate cortex (euphoria, fits) and the amygdala (fear). It is therefore possible that some of the more unusual kinds of acupuncture effects may be mediated by the limbic system (Campbell, 1999).

The role of neurotransmitters

A large number of neurotransmitters is known to exist but the relevance of most of them to acupuncture is uncertain. When acupuncture began to attract attention from researchers in the 1970s much importance was attached to the opioid peptides, which seemed to provide a ready explanation for acupuncture analgesia. Three classes of opioids are involved in analgesia: enkephalins, beta-endorphin, and dynorphin. Low-frequency electroacupuncture triggers release of beta-endorphin and enkephalin in the brain and spinal cord, whereas high-frequency electroacupuncture increases the release of dynorphin in the spinal cord. There has been much controversy about the relevance of the endogenous opioids to acupuncture analgesia and the position is still unclear.

One paradoxical finding is that stimuli that produce release of opioid peptides also cause release of an antagonist to them: cholecystokinin. It has been suggested that the ineffectiveness of acupuncture in about 20 per cent of the population may be related to higher than usual secretion rates of cholecystokinin.

Serotonin has been shown in some experiments to increase the effectiveness of acupuncture analgesia.

Oxytocin is another possible candidate for a role in acupuncture. It is released centrally in response to suckling. In rats, it causes analgesia. It appears to cause feelings of calm and relaxation in humans, and these commonly occur in patients receiving acupuncture.

Can peripheral stimulation modify the function of the central nervous system?

Critics sometimes say that it is absurd to suppose that insertion of a small needle into the body could produce far-reaching effects. However, there is now experimental evidence to show that this does indeed occur. Today it is increasingly being recognized that the adult nervous system is much more plastic than was supposed even a few years ago, and the possibility that it can be substantially remapped and reorganized by peripheral stimulation no longer seems far-fetched. The following study is relevant.

Cortical remapping by peripheral stimulation

Normal volunteers were given tactile stimulation to the right lower lip and simultaneously received painful electrical stimulation to the right median nerve (Knecht et al., 1998). When the tactile stimulation to the lip was repeated on its own, the volunteers again felt the sensation at the wrist, and one girl actually felt as if her fist were clenched. This experiment shows that even brief painful stimulation can bring about significant changes in central sensory mapping. The feeling of a clenched fist is quite often reported by patients with phantom limbs, and it may be that after amputation of an arm, say, the shoulder may be stimulated abnormally and may 'expand' into the now silenced arm map.

Referred itch

We should also remember that the central connections of the nervous system are a good deal more complex than is often recognized. This is evident from the phenomenon of referred itch (sometimes known by its German name *Mitempfindungen*). Evans, a neurologist, published an interesting paper (Evans, 1976) on this. About one person in four or five finds that scratching an irritation may produce an itch elsewhere. The sensation is well localized, comes and goes quickly, and recurs when scratching is repeated a short time later. The referral is to the same side as that scratched. The referral isn't reciprocal; that is, scratching the site of referred itch doesn't cause the original spot to itch. Different people don't necessarily have the same patterns of referral. Scratching the face, soles, or palms doesn't produce the effect. The mechanism of this phenomenon is unknown, though one suggestion is that it may be thalamic.

Acupuncture: art or science?

In emphasizing the scientific aspects of modern acupuncture, I'm in danger of overlooking the very real sense in which it is also partly an art. It may indeed depend on neurophysiological processes, but it also depends on manual skill that has to be learned, and it's here that some of the conceptual difficulties become most pronounced. How the acupuncture is actually performed affects the outcome. Some therapists get better results than others. This is a potentially damaging admission, which may seem to be tantamount to bringing in the much-derided 'good bedside manner' and to acknowledging that the whole of acupuncture is due to the placebo effect after all.

The answer, I think, is that the placebo concept means one thing in the context of drug trials but another when applied to manual therapies such as acupuncture. I return to this subject in Part 4, where I discuss acupuncture research in more detail; here I want to say only that the debate about whether the effects of needling are 'merely placebo' seems rather to miss the point. We actually know very little about what the placebo effect is, but there seems to be a widespread impression that it is somehow unreal, and therefore disreputable. But this must be wrong. Unless you are a Cartesian dualist, who believes in a separate mind hovering over the body, the placebo effect must ultimately be a neurophysiological phenomenon (Campbell, 1994). It must depend on brain states. And there is no difficulty, surely, in allowing that changes in brain state influence those areas, such as the limbic system, hypothalamus, and brain stem, that are concerned with pain perception as well as with endocrine and immune functioning. Thus, information, both verbal and non-verbal (needle-mediated), will be expected to have an important effect on how the body functions.

In fact, this process may not be confined to the needling itself. In the course of an acupuncture consultation there is both verbal and non-verbal interaction between therapist and patient, much of it at an unconscious level. Acupuncture is a thoroughly manual technique, and even before the actual needling begins the therapist will very probably have carried out a manual examination of the patient, checking the joints for range of movement, the muscles for tenderness and tone, and so forth. This process is, I suspect, therapeutic in itself, independently of the needling, which may account for the feeling that acupuncturists sometimes report that 'something is transmitted' via the needles. Nothing is transmitted in that sense, but information is certainly communicated by the entire acupuncture procedure (Campbell, 2000).

It may reassure the traditionalists if I say that even modern acupuncture, as I see it, is to a considerable extent an intuitive affair. The underlying theory of the modern approach is derived from modern anatomy, neurophysiology, pathology, and so on, but the treatment itself is still a person-to-person encounter that relies on the sense of touch to a great extent. (This is one reason why I generally dislike the use of electrical stimulation and so-called point detection with electrical apparatus.) As a manual technique, acupuncture runs counter to the general trend of medicine today.

Nowadays we are so well served by diagnostic methods such as computed tomography, magnetic resonance imaging, and other technological marvels that it's hardly necessary for doctors to examine their patients physically. Why guess what's happening inside a patient's body by tapping and pressing and listening, when you can actually see inside in astonishing detail? Treatment, too, is largely technological, using drugs, lasers, ultrasound, and other gifts of science. Yet manual treatments still are used and still are valuable, though it is mainly physiotherapists, osteopaths, and chiropractors who go in for these. Physiotherapist friends tell me that some years ago they were relying to a considerable extent on electrical machinery of various kinds, but in recent years they have increasingly reverted to manual therapies, which they find more effective. Doctors who wish to practise acupuncture will have to follow their physiotherapist colleagues in that direction.

Summary and conclusions

There is now a reasonable body of research to explain, at least in outline, how acupuncture might produce pain relief. However, we are certainly a long way from being able to supply a complete explanation of acupuncture analgesia. For one thing, much of the experimental work has been done on animals and, for another, most of it is concerned with short-term pain relief. Nevertheless, the research that has been carried out to date is enough to move acupuncture from the realm of fantasy to that of serious science.

References

Bowsher D. (1998) Mechanisms of acupuncture. In: *Medical Acupuncture* (eds Filshie J., White A.). Churchill Livingstone, Edinburgh.

Campbell A. (1994) Cartesian dualism and the concept of medical placebos. *Journal of Consciousness Studies*, 1; 230–3.

Campbell A. (1999) The limbic system and emotion in relation to acupuncture. *Acupuncture in Medicine*, 17; 124–30.

Campbell A. (2000) Acupuncture, touch and the placebo response. *Complementary Therapies in Medicine*, 8; 43–6.

Devor M. (1995) Pain networks. In: *The Handbook of Brain Theory and Neural Networks* (ed. Arbib M.A.). The MIT Press, Cambridge (Massachusetts), London (England).

Ernst E. & White A. (eds) (1999) *Acupuncture: a scientific appraisal*. Butterworth-Heinemann, Oxford.

Evans P.R. (1976) Referred itch (*Mitempfindungen*). *British Medical Journal*, 2; 839–41.

Han J.S. (1987) Mesolimbic neuronal loop of analgesia. In: *Advances in Pain Research and Therapy* (eds Tiengo M., Eccles J., Cuello A.C. & Ottoson D.), Vol 10. Raven Press, New York.

Knecht S., Sörus P., Günther, *et al.* (1998) Phantom sensations following acute pain. *Pain*, 77; 209–13.

Wall P.D. (2000) *The Science of Pain and Suffering*. Weidenfeld & Nicolson, London.

Wall, P.D. & Melzack, R. (eds) (1984) *A Textbook of Pain*. Churchill Livingstone, Edinburgh.

Part 2

Chapter 4

Risks of acupuncture

A knowledge of the potential risks of acupuncture is obviously the most essential thing that any would-be acupuncturist must acquire. One shouldn't exaggerate the dangers; acupuncture is generally remarkably safe if performed responsibly by someone with an adequate knowledge of anatomy. To put this in perspective, the risks in performing acupuncture are probably less than those of giving a conventional non-steroidal anti-inflammatory drug (NSAID). Nevertheless, it is an invasive procedure and this means that certain dangers are inevitably present (Hagen & Peukar, 1999). Most are relevant to the patient, but some apply to the person carrying out the treatment, who is at risk of needle-stick injury.

Infection

Bacterial infections

Bacterial infections are very rare indeed provided disposable needles are used. The needles should not, of course, be inserted through areas of skin that are obviously infected. Needles should also not be inserted into joint cavities unless full antiseptic precautions are taken, but this form of treatment is in any case unnecessary and undesirable.

The main exception to the statement that bacterial infection is not a threat concerns the use of press needles that are left in place for long periods, mainly in the ear. These can certainly cause local infections. In the case of the ear these may take the form of perichondritis, which is difficult to treat and may result in distortion of the auricle.

A more serious complication of using these needles is bacterial endocarditis. This has occurred in a number of cases. In my view, the risk makes it undesirable to use prolonged needling of this kind except perhaps in patients who are in hospital.

There are other arguments against using indwelling needles in the ear. It is possible that they may fall out and perhaps injure someone else; they could also, theoretically, fall into the ear canal, though I have not heard of this happening.

Viral infections

The main viral infection that may be transmitted by acupuncture is hepatitis B. (Hepatitis C has not so far been reported, perhaps because it has not been recognized for long enough.) Human immunodeficiency virus (HIV) could also theoretically be transmitted, but so far there are no proved cases of this. There are, however, numerous cases of hepatitis B transmission. There is a high incidence of hepatitis B in China and some people suspect that acupuncture is partly to blame for this.

Viral infection of patients is prevented by using disposable needles. The risk to the acupuncturist from needle-stick injuries is discussed further in Chapter 5. People practising acupuncture should be immunized against hepatitis B.

Patients who are blood donors require a letter to state that any acupuncture treatment they have received was carried out by a suitably trained health professional using disposable needles; without this they will be rejected as donors.

Haemorrhage

Minor capillary bleeding after acupuncture is quite common but is generally insignificant and can be controlled by local pressure with a swab. Sometimes a small swelling appears just after the needle is withdrawn; this is due to a haematoma. It should be flattened with local pressure to stop the bleeding and make the swelling absorb more quickly. Sometimes a local bruise appears at the site of needling, though it may not be apparent until some time later; patients should be warned about this possibility since otherwise they may be alarmed.

Patients who are taking anticoagulants or anti-platelet drugs are obviously in more danger of bleeding. This includes low-dose aspirin, which patients may take without necessarily consulting their doctor. All drugs of this kind are therefore at least a relative contraindication to acupuncture. However, superficial acupuncture (subcutaneous only) is probably safe, but deep (intramuscular) acupuncture, periosteal acupuncture, and acupuncture in the muscular compartments in the arm and leg should definitely be avoided.

Needle fracture

This is unlikely but not impossible. Good-quality disposable needles are generally reliable but should not be inserted 'up to the hilt', since the finer kinds tend to bend at this point. If a needle should break, an attempt should be made to pull it out with sterile forceps; if this fails, the patient will have to go to a hospital casualty department. 'Jumping' when the needle is inserted is most likely to cause a break. To avoid this, always warn the patient before inserting a needle.

Fainting

As with any other minor surgical procedure, including venesection and injections, patients may faint when receiving acupuncture. Young fit men are particularly likely to do this. Very apprehensive patients of either sex and any age may faint but these are in any case unsuitable for acupuncture, as it is likely to be ineffective. If a patient is thought likely to faint, they should be placed in a suitable position so that they don't slide onto the floor.

Sweating

Patients receiving acupuncture may sweat profusely. Often this may be a manifestation of anxiety, but not always. Some people routinely sweat when needled, especially in the hands, even though they don't appear to be anxious.

Convulsions

Occasionally patients receiving acupuncture have an epileptic fit. This is certainly uncommon: in over 25 years' practice I have never seen a case, but it has been reported a number of times. It is generally attributed to cerebral anoxia, since it has usually, though not exclusively, occurred when patients were treated sitting rather than lying down, and is then thought to be a complication of fainting. However, I have a suspicion that there may be another factor involved. The limbic system, and especially the anterior cingulate cortex, are areas that are often implicated in the genesis of epilepsy of various kinds (Campbell, 1999). There is a good deal of evidence to suggest that acupuncture activates the limbic system, and this may be an additional reason why seizures may occur.

Fits of this kind generally don't occur in people with a history of previous epileptic attacks and should not be taken as necessarily indicating an epileptic tendency in other circumstances.

Miscarriage

There are numerous anecdotal reports of miscarriage occurring in patients receiving acupuncture, especially in the first three months of pregnancy. Miscarriage is common so the association may be simply due to chance, but it's best to assume that there is a causal connection. Acupuncture is therefore contraindicated in pregnancy unless there is a strong reason for it to be done. The commonest such reason is severe vomiting in pregnancy. Many doctors are currently using the anti-nausea site in the wrist (PC6) to treat this, and report good results, and it appears to be safe. There are certain 'forbidden areas' in pregnancy: the abdomen, the lower back, and the 'spleen' areas in the lower limbs (SP6, SP9, SP10), which are related to the pelvic organs in women. Strong stimulation at any site should always be avoided in pregnancy.

Drowsiness

Some degree of relaxation is common after acupuncture. In some people this goes on to become frank drowsiness. There is thus a risk that patients will be unsafe if driving or operating machinery after acupuncture. (I knew one man who drove the wrong way round a roundabout.) Patients should therefore be advised not to drive a car after receiving acupuncture; if this is unavoidable they should be warned to take extra care and this should be recorded in the case notes.

The risk is greatest after the first treatment but may occur every time or may not be seen until several treatments have been given. The onset of sleepiness is not necessarily immediate; it may occur some hours later.

Anatomical damage

This is the most serious risk attached to acupuncture. Probably almost every organ in the body has been pierced by an acupuncturist at some time or other, but the commonest lesion is pneumothorax.

Pneumothorax

This may be fatal. Patients with reduced pulmonary function, and those who suffer a tension pneumothorax, are at particular risk of dying. Needling anywhere over the chest wall is capable of causing pneumothorax and another important danger site is the trapezius muscle (GB21) or other areas above the clavicle. It is important to realize that the symptoms and signs of pneumothorax (shortness of breath, decreased breath sounds, increased resonance to percussion, and so on) may not appear until 24 hours have elapsed; X-ray changes may also not be seen immediately. If pneumothorax occurs or is suspected the patient must be sent urgently to a hospital casualty department.

Cardiac tamponade

This occurs when bleeding into the pericardial sac compromises the pumping action of the heart; it is fatal if untreated. At least six cases caused by acupuncture have been reported. In these cases the needle penetrated the sternum through a congenital defect called the foramen sternale, which occurs in about 5–8 per cent of the population. There is a frequently used classic acupuncture in this region (CV17). The defect is not reliably detectable by palpation or radiography. Needling over the sternum should therefore always be done tangentially and superficially. (I find there is generally little benefit from using this site and seldom do so.)

Spinal cord

The spinal cord is at risk when patients are needled over the vertebrae. The distance from the skin to the spinal cord or the roots of the spinal nerves varies from 25 mm to 45 mm in different patients. The spinal cord is said to terminate at the lower border of L1 in adults, but, like most anatomical norms, this is somewhat variable. There are classic acupuncture points in the neck (especially GV14 and GV15) that are potentially dangerous for the spinal cord and brain stem. Again, there is seldom any good reason to needle these sites in modern acupuncture practice.

Abdominal organs

Any abdominal organ (liver, spleen, stomach, intestines, urinary bladder, kidneys, etc.) is potentially at risk. The risk is greater if the organ in question is enlarged for any reason.

Eye and orbit

There are several classic acupuncture points in the neighbourhood of the eye and orbit and these need special care.

Injury to peripheral nerves

Peripheral nerves are quite often touched during acupuncture and this gives rise to pain like an electric shock, which is generally evanescent and not serious but may at times be long-lasting. I know of one doctor who was needled during a training course at LI4 in the hand; he had pain in the thumb after this which lasted for six months before finally resolving. A case of foot drop caused by needling the fibular nerve at ST36 has been reported, and so has a case of bilateral hand swelling following acupuncture to LI4 (see Chapter 15).

Forgotten needles

It is easy to forget to remove a needle, especially in patients with long hair if this conceals needles inserted in the neck or over the shoulders. Ways of preventing this are discussed below.

Electrical stimulation

This can inhibit or derange the function of a demand pacemaker. Electroacupuncture should not be applied to any patient fitted with such a pacemaker.

Allergic reactions to needles

It is recommended that patients who are allergic to particular metals such as chromium or zinc should not be treated. In practice, allergic reactions are seldom seen.

Miscellaneous

The foregoing headings do not cover all the adverse effects that have been attributed to acupuncture, though they do include the main ones. There are numerous methods of performing acupuncture and some of those used, particularly in Japan, have special risks attached. It is not always easy to tell, from published reports, whether the adverse effects experienced were really due to acupuncture.

General precautions when performing acupuncture

The dangers of acupuncture, especially the risks of anatomical damage, make it essential that this treatment should be performed only by people who have been adequately trained. Anatomy is obviously of particular importance but different kinds of health professionals employ anatomical knowledge to differing extents in their ordinary work. The everyday practice of clinical medicine does not always require detailed knowledge of anatomy.

When performing acupuncture in a potentially hazardous anatomical region you should make sure your anatomical knowledge is fresh and adequate. If there is any doubt in your mind you should either not do acupuncture at all or else confine yourself to superficial needling no deeper than the subcutaneous tissues; this is safe and may be surprisingly effective. Remember, it's never compulsory to perform acupuncture!

Two classes of patient require particular care: those who are very obese, because the anatomical landmarks may be difficult or impossible to identify, and those who are very thin, because the distance from the skin to vital organs is short.

Safety precautions

The following safety precautions are designed to minimize the risk of needle-stick injury, an ever-present danger for the acupuncturist.

- Students are often taught that they can use the same needle in a number of sites on the same patient. This is acceptable so far as risk to the patient is concerned, not so for the acupuncturist. Each time you insert a needle there is a small but not negligible risk that you will prick your other hand. It is much preferable to do this with an unused needle. I therefore advise students to use each needle once only.
- It is generally said that, in withdrawing a needle, you should steady the skin with the opposite hand. This creates a small risk that, as you withdraw the needle, you will prick the steadying hand. I therefore advise taking needles out with one hand, keeping the other hand well clear.
- As soon as the needle is withdrawn it should be disposed of in the 'sharps' bin, before any conversation with the patient or onlookers begins, and before starting to write notes. In disposing of the needle, avoid putting it point first into the bin, because the tip may catch on the edge of the aperture, causing the needle to fly through the air. Needles should be held horizontally above the bin and dropped in from a short distance.

Avoid forgetting needles

One way of avoiding forgetting to remove needles is to insert only one needle at a time. In this way, you withdraw each needle before inserting the next and there is no chance of forgetting one. This way of practising is easy to do for the sort of acupuncture I mostly use, in which only a few needles are inserted and they are left in for brief periods. It is less suitable for practitioners who insert large numbers of needles or who leave them in for longer periods. Alternatively, keep a count of the needles inserted and this can be compared with the number of empty needle packages. Finally, make a quick visual and manual check of the area.

Surface anatomy

See Chapter 12, pp. 121–122 for details of surface anatomy in the thoracic and lumbar regions.

References

Campbell A. (1999) The limbic system and emotion in relation to acupuncture. *Acupuncture in Medicine*, 17; 124–30.

Hagen R. & Peukar E. (1999). Adverse effects of acupuncture. In: *Acupuncture: a scientific appraisal* (eds Ernst E. & White A.). Butterworth-Heinemann, Oxford.

Chapter 5

Principles of treatment

By definition, acupuncture consists in the use of needles. Injection needles are not suitable for this purpose, for various reasons: they have a cutting edge which makes them more liable to damage structures such as blood vessels and nerves, they are hollow and therefore, at least theoretically, more likely to introduce infection, and they do not produce the typical acupuncture sensations known as de qi. Proper acupuncture needles should therefore always be used.

Formerly, needles were reused many times. They were cleaned and sterilized and sometimes they were sharpened on a stone to remove the small hooks that tended to form at their tips. With increasing awareness of the risk of transmitting infections such as hepatitis and HIV, however, this is no longer acceptable, and only disposable needles should now be used. Thanks to this change in practice, disposable needles have become widely available and are quite inexpensive; they are also better in quality than they used to be.

Types of needles

The needles in common use have a shaft and a handle, so that they somewhat resemble a small rapier. Previously the handle was made of fine wire wound round the needle: this type is still available, but there are also needles whose handles are made of plastic. These are equally satisfactory provided electrical stimulation is not needed. The shaft of the needle is normally made of steel; gold and silver needles are also available and are said by some to have special properties, but there is no good evidence for this.

Other types of needles exist. Very short needles are used to treat the ear; these are shaped like small drawing pins made of wire and project only about 1 mm into the skin. They can be used in other locations than the ear when very superficial stimulation is required. Practitioners of traditional acupuncture sometimes use a 'plum blossom hammer'; this is a mallet with short needles set in its face, which allows scarification of the skin over an area. Sterilization of these instruments is difficult.

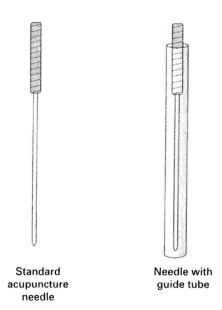

Standard
acupuncture
needle

Needle with
guide tube

Types of needles

Needles may be supplied with a guide tube or 'introducer'. This is a plastic tube in which the needle is lightly fixed. The tube is slightly shorter than the needle so that the tip of the handle projects above the top of the tube, where it may be held in place by a little plastic wedge. To insert the needle, the operator places the tip of the tube against the skin, removes the wedge (if present) and taps the end of the handle to drive the needle about 2 mm into the skin. The tube is then removed and the needle is advanced to the desired depth.

Beginners are often taught to use these tubes. Many experienced acupuncturists, including me, dislike them and remove them before inserting the needles. It is a matter of choice whether or not to use the tubes, but if you are dependent on them you may encounter difficulties if the only needles available happen to lack them. I don't like to teach people to use techniques I don't use myself and I therefore always show students how to insert the plain needles, but there is no reason why acupuncturists should not use the tubes if they wish. One advantage of using them is that the pressure of the tube appears to act as a distraction and makes the penetration of the needle almost painless. This is sometimes given as a reason for using them, since it is said to make treating apprehensive patients easier; but acupuncture generally doesn't work in apprehensive patients, so it is usually better not to treat them at all.

Regardless of whether tubes are used or not, the needles should be packed individually, since otherwise it is difficult to extract one or two needles without rendering others unsterile.

Lengths and thicknesses

Needles come in varying lengths and thicknesses. The most useful needle is 30–40 mm in length and either 0.25 mm or 0.30 mm in diameter. The thicker needles are easier to insert but more painful for the patient. Shorter needles are 15 mm in length and are also thinner, either 0.15 or 0.20 mm in diameter. These are useful when shallow insertion, with more gentle stimulation, is desired. Longer needles are needed for deep needling, for example over the lower back; for this, needles 50 mm in length are often used. They need to be fairly stout (0.30 mm) since otherwise they will be difficult to insert. Still longer needles are available and may on occasion be needed to reach deep structures such as the piriformis muscle.

Using the needles

The technique of inserting the needles is simple but requires practice if it is to be done skilfully and relatively painlessly. Acquiring good needle technique is an important part of achieving success in acupuncture. It is customary to begin by needling oranges, but these don't give the same sensation as needling patients. A better simulation can be achieved by

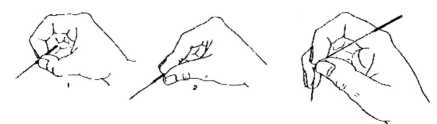

Techniques for inserting needles

placing a piece of thin card over the orange and needling through this. A still better plan is to practise on oneself (see Chapter 19). This has two advantages: one learns exactly what the patient is going to experience and there is an excellent incentive to avoid overstimulation!

In what follows I describe the process of needle insertion in a number of steps. This is to some extent artificial, since in practice the needle is inserted in a smooth continuous action, but it is convenient to analyse it in this way in order to clarify how it works.

A. Preliminaries

● The patient needs to be positioned properly. The details vary according to the area to be treated; this will be discussed later (in Part 3) in connection with treatment of the different anatomical areas. However, the general principle is that the muscles need to be put under slight stretch.

- The acupuncturist should wash his or her hands. This is important because, as I shall explain, it is often inevitable that the shaft of the needle be supported manually during insertion.
- The patient is warned that the needle is about to be inserted, otherwise he or she may jump and bend or even break the needle. I usually say 'Needle going in now'.

B. Insertion (the description assumes a right-handed operator)

- Stretch the skin with the left hand.
- Rest the tip of the needle against the skin. (Alternatively, place the tip of the guide tube against the skin.)
- Press the tip of the needle right through the skin, without hesitating. (Alternatively, tap the end of the handle to force the needle tip through the skin.)
- Advance the needle to the desired depth (see discussion of 'depth' below).
- Wait and assess response (about 15 seconds). This means: keep asking the patient what they are feeling. Say 'What do you feel?'; don't ask 'Does it hurt?' Inquire about general effects as well as local effects. Watch the patient's face, not the needle site. If there is continuing pain after the needle is inserted, remove it at once.
- If stimulation is required, twist or 'peck' (if needling the periosteum). Again, wait and assess the response.
- If necessary, repeat the stimulation.
- Withdraw the needle and dispose of it safely.

Duration of needling

This whole process takes between 10 seconds and two minutes, which is very considerably less than the 20 minutes generally used by traditional practitioners and also less than the 20–30 minutes advised by some modern acupuncturists who base their recommendation on physiological considerations. It may seem surprising that such brief needling is effective, but in practice it is, difficult though that may be to explain. One possible reason why it works is that the nervous system adapts very quickly to a new stimulus and soon ceases to register it. Also, although the needle is withdrawn quickly it must leave a small area of traumatized tissue which presumably will continue to send impulses into the spinal cord for a considerable time afterwards – certainly for some hours,

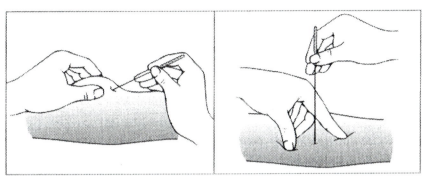

Techniques for manipulating needles

probably for some days. In any case, experience amply demonstrates that this type of needling is clinically effective, and indeed there seem to be some patients who will only respond to acupuncture if it is done in this way. (See 'minimalist acupuncture', below.)

Some alternative techniques

The skin may be surprisingly hard to penetrate. In that case, the needle may be twisted as it is inserted, with a drill-like action, or it may be 'bounced' through the skin with a series of little thrusts.

If the skin is resistant the needle will tend to bend, especially if a guide tube is not used. To prevent this, the acupuncturist needs to squeeze the needle firmly between finger and thumb, and may need to grip the shaft some way below the handle (hence the need for scrupulously clean hands).

Longer needles, such as the 50 mm needle, require a different technique for insertion, since they tend to wobble about unduly. The most convenient method is to flex the needle with the middle finger so that it is effectively shortened (again, clean hands are essential). The 'bouncing' technique, described above, may be useful here.

The short 15 mm needles, being relatively flimsy, may bend at the junction between the shaft and handle. For this reason they should not be inserted 'up to the hilt'. Apart from this, however, they are easy to insert.

Students sometimes ask if they should swab the skin before inserting the needle. The evidence that this makes any difference to the chance of infection is scanty and the weight of opinion these days is that it is unnecessary, although it may be advisable if the skin is visibly dirty. If you apply alcohol, allow enough time for it to evaporate before inserting the needle, otherwise the patient will experience stinging.

Depth of needling

Beginners often ask how deeply they should needle. The obvious, if unhelpful, answer is: 'as deep as necessary'. That is, if you want to needle a particular muscle, or the periosteum, you will have to go down to the relevant depth. In other cases, more superficial needling is appropriate. Naturally, the anatomy must be kept in mind; there is much more depth of tissue in the gluteal region, for example, than in the face, and such differences will affect how deeply the needles are inserted. We frequently compress the tissues with the free hand in order to reduce the depth that the needle has to penetrate.

The possible depths of needling are as follows:

- intradermal
- subcutaneous
- intramuscular
- periosteal/ligamentous

Intradermal acupuncture, in which the needle just enters the dermis, should be avoided because it is both painful and relatively ineffectual. Any of the other depths may be needed, depending on the site to be needled, the disorder being treated, and other factors.

The most sensitive tissues are the skin and the periosteum. Once the skin has been penetrated, advancing the needle further generally does not cause much pain or other sensation until the periosteum is reached.

Minimalist acupuncture (micro-acupuncture – Mann)

This is a very gentle form of acupuncture, in which the needle is inserted only as far as the subcutaneous tissue and withdrawn after a few seconds with little or no manual stimulation. Although it might seem so gentle a treatment as to be without effect, the contrary is the case, and there are some patients who will only respond to this form of needling. Mann uses this technique extensively and a number of practitioners, including me, have independently moved in that direction to some extent. This brings us to the very interesting question of 'dosification'.

'Dosification' in acupuncture

This an important subject. In fact, I would almost go so far as to say that the 'quantity' of stimulus is more important than the exact site at which it's applied. The general principle is to use the minimal stimulation possible, particularly on the first occasion. It is easy to over-treat a patient, difficult to under-treat. There is a natural tendency to feel that, if a certain stimulus is effective, using a stronger stimulus will be still more effective, but this doesn't seem to be the case in acupuncture. There are just a few patients who seem to need strong stimulation for the treatment to work, whereas there are many who will only respond to gentle stimulation. Treating such people too strongly may not only cause severe aggravations, but also often fails to produce any therapeutic effect at all.

Strength of stimulus increases with:

1. the number of needles used;
2. the thickness of the needles;
3. the amount of stimulation (twisting or 'pecking').

The depth of needling is less important, unless the periosteum is reached, in which case the stimulation becomes stronger. So to achieve gentle stimulation, use a fine needle, twist it little or not at all, and reduce the time it is left in place; this can be as little as half a second, incredible though that may seem.

Effects of acupuncture

Once the needle is inserted a number of things may happen.

1. Local effects
   - You may feel a resistance to twirling the needle. What produces this effect is not known, but it is a common finding and is sometimes called 'muscle grasp'. It can be surprisingly strong and may make it impossible to withdraw the needle at first. If so, wait for a few minutes and then try again. Some books say that one can release a 'caught' needle by inserting another needle a short distance away, but this is seldom necessary.
   The patient may feel a variety of sensations produced by acupuncture for a variable distance round the needle. These are usually difficult to describe. They may travel up or down the limb; occasionally they are felt in distant parts of the body. All these phenomena, those experienced by you, the acupuncturist, and those experienced by the patient, are collectively called de qi. Traditionalists attach a great deal of importance to it and indeed often say that it is essential for a good therapeutic response. This is an overstatement, but de qi probably does mean that a good response is more likely. In needling muscle trigger points it seems to be an indication that the needle has reached the right spot.
2. General effects
   - A certain degree of relaxation is so common with acupuncture as to be almost the rule. In some people this is more pronounced and reaches the stage of drowsiness. There may also be euphoria; patients may compare this to the effects of alcohol or hashish. These

very interesting effects may possibly be due to endorphin release, although against this idea is the fact that they come on surprisingly quickly, often almost as soon as the needle is inserted. This suggests the possibility that they are due to limbic system effects, since some parts of this system, notably the anterior cingulate cortex, may produce euphoria when stimulated (Campbell, 1999). If they are marked they suggest that the patient is a strong reactor (see below).

Response variations in acupuncture patients

There is a wide range of responses to acupuncture in different patients. At one extreme, some do not respond at all, while at the other extreme some experience a profound effect. In rough terms the picture is as follows:

- 20 per cent: no response
- 60 per cent: average response
- 20 per cent: strong or very strong response

Strong reactors

It is important to recognize the group who respond strongly, because they are the easiest to help with acupuncture but also the easiest to make worse by over-treatment. The existence of this group of strong responders seems to have been recognized first by Mann. He gives certain characteristics that help one to recognize strong responders before they are treated: they may be particularly sensitive to art or to natural beauty, and they may give a history of intolerance to a range of prescribed medications. The ability to recognize potential strong responders also develops with experience. After treating a wide range of patients with acupuncture for some years one begins to categorize them, subconsciously, as corresponding to certain types. In this way it becomes possible to predict, with reasonable accuracy, who will and who will not respond well to acupuncture; but there are always surprises.

When treated, strong responders experience marked general effects. They are particularly likely to become euphoric or may feel as if they have taken alcohol or other sorts of recreational drugs, if they are familiar with these. They may also experience marked radiation effects, so that, for example, a needle inserted in the foot may cause feelings of warmth in the chest or face, sometimes accompanied by flushing. The effects of acupuncture in such cases can be striking and unexpected.

Some patients experience emotional abreactions during or just after receiving acupuncture. These may take the form of crying or laughing. Some people find themselves giggling at everything that is said, whether or not it is facetious. Many though not all patients who react in this way will be strong responders.

Patients who have had acupuncture on a previous occasion sometimes report that it was a very unpleasant experience and they felt very ill for some time afterwards. Such people are nearly always strong responders who were treated too vigorously, with large numbers of needles being inserted and left in for 20 minutes or more, perhaps with electrical stimulation. If they are treated very gently, with perhaps just one or two needles which are inserted and removed almost immediately, they generally do very well.

Pseudo-strong responders

I have seen a number of patients whom I would classify in this category although I have not seen it described anywhere. They generally arrive for treatment with protestations of belief in acupuncture and convey a sense of expectation and enthusiasm. The first time they are treated they usually have a dramatic response, with euphoria and other effects resembling those of a genuine strong responder. However, on the next occasion they have little or no response, and thereafter they become non-responders. A genuine strong responder, in contrast, will experience much the same effect at every treatment.

Belief status and response

Whether the patient believes in acupuncture before being treated seems to make no difference to the outcome. Indeed, scepticism is often a good sign, whereas strong belief sometimes suggests that a patient may be a pseudo-strong responder. However, fear of acupuncture is definitely a contra-indication to treatment, since it usually inhibits the response.

Response patterns in acupuncture

In general terms, only three things can happen when acupuncture is performed: the patient gets better, gets worse, or stays the same.

No change

As noted above, about 20 per cent of the population appears not to respond to acupuncture at all. This figure has emerged from the majority of clinical trials of acupuncture done in the West. The likelihood that a given patient will be in this category increases rapidly if no improvement has occurred after two or three treatments, and it is seldom worthwhile continuing beyond this stage. Exceptions to this rule do occur, but it takes considerable experience to know when it is worth continuing longer, perhaps trying different approaches. Certainly there is no case for carrying out prolonged treatments in the face of non-response.

Improvement

This may be immediate or delayed. Some patients report an immediate relief of pain or increase in range of movement as soon as the needles are inserted. This is gratifying, of course, but it pays to be cautious, because sometimes these rapid improvements disappear as quickly as they came.

A more common effect is improvement that is delayed for some hours or days. Delayed improvement of this kind is generally more long-lasting than instantaneous improvement. Delays of two or three days are not unusual. Occasionally patients report that nothing happened for perhaps ten days and then they became much better; they may be kind enough to ascribe this to the acupuncture, but it seems more likely that they have experienced a spontaneous remission.

Aggravation

This refers to a temporary worsening of the existing symptoms. Minor aggravations are quite common; probably about 20 per cent of those who respond will experience temporary worsening to some degree. Provided the acupuncture is done gently such aggravations are seldom severe and most patients take them in their stride, especially if they are told that their occurrence is generally a favourable sign, which it is.

Aggravations can be reduced although not entirely eliminated by gentle treatment. If they are severe the advice generally given is to repeat the original treatment very gently, but in practice this is hardly ever necessary; most patients respond to reassurance.

Occasionally patients can only be made worse; no improvement follows the aggravation, no matter how lightly they are treated.

Repetition of treatment

Although some patients experience permanent relief of their symptoms after treatment (exceptionally after only one session), there are many who need repeated treatments at intervals to maintain remission. In chronic disease a typical pattern might be as follows.

Treatment 1: There is some relief of symptoms, with or without a preceding aggravation. This relief may last just a few days, possibly even less.

Treatment 2: (1–2 weeks later): This produces better or more prolonged relief.

Treatment 3: (2 weeks later): Still better relief, more prolonged.

Treatment 4: (4 weeks later): Patient now symptom-free much of the time.

Treatment 5: (4 weeks later): Little further change.

Treatment 6: (4 weeks later): Still no further change; patient is treated once more and asked to return if and when the symptoms seem to be getting worse.

Note that the second treatment is given 1 or 2 weeks after the first. It is not given before a week has elapsed because it is impossible to judge the effect of the first treatment before this. In acute disease, this interval could be shortened, but even then the second treatment should not be given until 2 or 3 days after the first.

In most cases, a 'plateau' of response is reached after approximately three to six treatments. We sometimes find recommendations to give longer courses of treatment, and six is said by some to be a minimum; however, there are undoubtedly patients who achieve an excellent response in fewer treatments.

Relief of symptoms may be complete, or there may be a partial but still worthwhile remission. It is probably not advisable to repeat the treatment while the patient is still on the 'plateau'; this means that some patients may not receive any treatment when they return for follow-up. In at least some cases, treating patients too soon may cause an aggravation.

Patients should be treated as and when they relapse. Ideally, this should be done as soon as the relapse begins, but in practice the results still seem to be good even if relapse is allowed to continue for quite a long time.

Brief relief of symptoms

Some patients experience good relief of symptoms but for only a short time, perhaps a week or so. When I first started practising acupuncture I used to get such people into hospital and treat them daily for about 10 days, in the hope that intensive acupuncture of this kind, which is apparently used in China, would give more prolonged relief. However, I never found that it did so.

If patients keep relapsing in this way one should search for precipitating factors. For example, are they sitting in an ergonomically unsatisfactory position at work, which is perpetuating their neck or back problems, or do they have a cat at home which is causing them to be asthmatic? If nothing of the kind is found, it may be possible for them to do their own acupuncture, but this depends on the site to be needled and other factors. (See Chapter 18 for details.)

There is no 'minimum' period for which acupuncture has to last before it is considered a success. Everything depends on the perceptions of the patient and the therapist. In some cases it may be practicable and satisfactory to treat someone every 4 weeks, say, to control their headaches. However, as a rule of thumb I tend to regard 8 weeks as the shortest worthwhile period of remission if acupuncture is to be continued over many months or even years.

Safety precautions

The precautions to prevent needle-stick injury to the operator, described in Chapter 4, should be observed.

References

Campbell A. (1998) Methods of acupuncture. In: *Medical Acupuncture: a Western scientific approach* (eds Filshie J. & White A.). Churchill Livingstone, Edinburgh.

Campbell A. (1999). The limbic system and emotion in relation to acupuncture. *Acupuncture in Medicine*, 17; 124–30.

Chapter 6

Choosing where to needle

In Chapter 5 I looked in some detail at the techniques of using the needles but I haven't said much about where they should be inserted. This usually seems to beginners to be the most important question. As experience increases, one begins to see that it may not be quite as important as it first appears; there seem to be almost as many opinions on the subject as there are acupuncturists, yet all claim much the same proportion of good responses. Critics may and do use this lack of specificity to dismiss the whole of acupuncture as based on illusion. The task is therefore to find a way of making sense of the apparent confusion in a way that will allow us to describe the treatment in a comprehensible matter. What I shall do in this chapter and the following is, first, to review the possible ways that exist for deciding where to place the needles. Next, I shall describe an approach to this difficult subject which, I believe, is a satisfactory one for practical purposes; this will provide me with the terminology I shall need in Part 3, where I give the details of the acupuncture treatments I use. Finally, I shall outline some general principles that will guide me in Part 3.

The present chapter and the succeeding one are in some ways the most important in the book, because they explain what I take to be the essence of modern acupuncture. If you are familiar with other ways of doing acupuncture you will see that this is a fairly radical approach, since it largely ignores the traditional apparatus of 'points'. Only a few of these are used, and then only in the sense that they provide a convenient shorthand description of needling sites. I do not want to claim that this is the 'right' way to view acupuncture, or the 'only' way, or the 'best' way. In other words, I don't say that I am the only man in step. The fact is that we don't know enough about the subject at present to make any such claims and it will be a long time before we can do so. At the moment, much of what is said about modern acupuncture, except for statements about safety, is based on personal opinion and experience. I do claim, however, that this way of doing acupuncture is at least as effective as any other, and is a lot easier to understand, and quicker to perform, than most others that I have come across.

With this disclaimer out of the way, we can get down to business. I start by reviewing the main ways of choosing where to insert the needles.

Traditional or traditional-derived methods

Traditional acupuncture, at least as currently described in the West, implies the full theory of qi, yin–yang polarity, points, and 'meridians'. It also requires the practitioner to adopt and use the ancient Chinese concepts of disease, which are difficult or impossible to equate with modern pathological concepts, and to practise obscure techniques such as pulse and tongue diagnosis. I have already pointed out (in Part 1) the problems that these entail.

The traditional system has also sprouted a number of offshoots that preserve some aspects of the original but depart from it in various ways. Examples are ear acupuncture (auriculotherapy), scalp acupuncture, and Ryodoraku (a Japanese system of electro-acupuncture). These derivative methods generally retain the concept of 'points' in some form and may also use a modified version of traditional pulse diagnosis. They could be called neoclassical acupuncture methods. I discuss some of them briefly in Part 4.

Because some Westerners wish to use the traditional system of points without immersing themselves in the full complexity of traditional theory, there exist 'cookbooks' that contain lists of sites to needle in different disorders. Beginners often find these attractive, but they suffer from the disadvantage that they provide no insight into what is happening. If the suggested treatment doesn't work, you are left with little idea of what to do next, apart from consulting a different cookbook. Another disadvantage of these books is that, because they generally list large numbers of points for each set of symptoms, they are liable to encourage over-treatment. Although it may seem tempting to rely on cookbooks, this should be resisted.

(In fact, the cooking metaphor is rather appropriate for acupuncture. When beginners learn to cook they generally follow the recipes in their cookbooks exactly, but they encounter difficulties if, for example, certain ingredients are lacking. Experienced cooks, in contrast, know the probable effects of mixing different ingredients together, and can substitute one for another. They can also make up variants on book recipes or even, on occasion, invent totally new dishes. Becoming a good cook depends, in part, on freeing oneself from undue dependence on books, although certain basic principles always apply. As I shall explain, acupuncture is much the same; you get to know the effect of treating certain areas and then apply this knowledge to the symptoms that patients complain of; in some cases this may result in apparently 'new' versions of treatment.)

Modern methods

The remaining methods of choosing where to needle are non-traditional; that is, they are attempts to reinterpret the basis of acupuncture in line with modern ideas of anatomy and physiology. We will look at four of these: segmental acupuncture; Gunn's radiculopathy approach; trigger point acupuncture, which is probably the most popular modern approach today; and Mann's version of modern acupuncture. I shall then put forward a descriptive terminology which, I hope, unites the best features of all the modern accounts.

Segmental acupuncture

It is well known that the nervous system has a segmental arrangement, a trait that we owe to our developmental origin from a primitive worm-like ancestor. This arrangement is the explanation for various patterns of referred pain, such as radiation down the arms in angina pectoris or sciatic radiation of pain down the leg. A spinal segment consists of a dermatome, a myotome, a sclerotome, and a viscerotome, located at the levels of the skin, muscle, bones and joints, and viscera, respectively. All these are interconnected by the same shared innervation and can influence one another. However, owing to the changes that occur during embryological development the various components of each segment don't usually overlap one another.

Many Western therapists who adopted acupuncture in the 1970s and 1980s thought that it could be explained in terms of the known segmental arrangement. Hence there has arisen what is called segmental acupuncture. The idea is intuitively appealing to an acupuncture modernist who wants to rationalize the procedure, since it seems to be firmly based on the known nervous system, but at the practical level it can be rather difficult to apply. One problem is that the segmental arrangement of the body itself, although undoubtedly correct in a general way, is not so fixed and clear-cut as the diagrams in textbooks might suggest. Another is that when segmental theory is applied to acupuncture a certain aura of vagueness and lack of precision begins to appear. Thus, we are told (Bekkering & van Bussel, 1998) that treatment may consist in needling a local point at the site of pain, a distant point in the disturbed dermatome, myotome, or sclerotome, a point in a dermatome, myotome, or sclerotome related to an affected organ, a point in a related segment, or a point in an unrelated segment with a separate problem that is acting as an aggravating factor. The student could be forgiven for concluding that almost any combination of treatment points could legitimately be described as coming under the rubric of segmental acupuncture.

In practice, acupuncture often works even when the site that is needled could not plausibly be related to a relevant spinal segment. This was vividly illustrated for me in a recent acupuncture training course.

A young woman had a needle inserted in GB21 on the left (C4 dermatome). Almost at once the whole of her left arm became flushed (C5–T1). After this had passed off a needle was inserted in her right cervical region (C3); this time the whole of her right arm became flushed. Phenomena like this indicate that the radiation from a needle may be much wider than that suggested by segmental considerations. The curious phenomenon of referred itch, mentioned in Chapter 3, is also relevant here.

As we shall see in a moment, the trigger point version of acupuncture uses referral patterns that are considerably wider than segmental theory would suggest. I conclude that it is a mistake to rely on this idea exclusively or even mainly; to this extent the traditional version of acupuncture, which assumes heterosegmental effects of needles, is correct. On the other hand, two acupuncture treatments that I use could be described as segmental. Inserting a needle directly into a painful area must obviously imply needling within the same spinal segment, and so, too, does periosteal acupuncture, in which one needles around the affected joint; this, too, is a form of segmental (sclerotomal) acupuncture. Segmental acupuncture, then, is part of the modern version of acupuncture, but by no means the whole story.

Radiculopathy approach (Gunn, 1998)

Most Western theorizing about acupuncture has focused on the central nervous system and on neurochemistry. A Canadian doctor, C.C. Gunn, thinks that this neglects the importance of the peripheral nervous system.

Gunn claims that acupuncture points are nearly always situated close to known neuroanatomic entities, such as muscle motor points (the site where the main motor nerve enters the muscle) or musculotendinous junctions. Effective treatment sites are said to lie mainly within the same segment or segments as those containing the patient's symptoms. There are usually palpable muscle bands at these sites, and the affected muscles are shortened by spasm and contracture. The symptoms and signs disappear when the tender and tight muscle bands are needled. As we shall see in the next section, this description corresponds exactly with standard descriptions of trigger points, but Gunn's theory differs in that he attributes these effects to 'radiculopathy', which, as he acknowledges, is not familiar as a clinical entity to all Western physicians, although it was first described a long time ago.

The theory holds that a peripheral nerve may appear normal and may continue to function, yet may cause a condition of 'supersensitivity' in which the structures supplied by the nerve behave abnormally. There are said to be innumerable causes of radiculopathy (trauma, inflammation, infection, metabolic, degenerative, toxic ...) but the commonest is probably spondylosis. Striated muscle is the structure most strongly affected by the disorder; the muscle in question becomes contracted, painful, and afflicted by trigger points. There may also be autonomic effects on viscera.

Gunn doesn't use the term acupuncture to describe his needling treatment, preferring to call it 'intramuscular stimulation' (IMS). He claims it is 'many times more effective' than traditional acupuncture.

I have some difficulty with Gunn's description of radiculopathy, which seems to be in some danger of falling into circularity. We are told that a nerve affected by this disorder produces changes in the muscles it supplies, but we are also told that the nerve in question may appear to be 'deceptively normal'. The muscle, however, behaves as if it were denervated. This means that the only way we can tell that a nerve is suffering from radiculopathy is by its effects on the muscle; but it was the effects on the muscle that the concept of radiculopathy was intended to explain in the first place.

However, if we leave this theoretical question aside, what are left with? Gunn's IMS seems to include segmental acupuncture and trigger point acupuncture but doesn't add much to them in a practical sense; it just offers an alternative explanation of how they work. On the practical level, the treatments he describes are much the same as those used by other non-traditional acupuncturists, although perhaps rather more vigorous. I have no doubt that they are effective, but I don't find the need to set acupuncture in this particular context.

Trigger point acupuncture (Baldry, 1998)

A number of Western writers on acupuncture have attached a lot of importance to the notion of trigger points; indeed, some think that the whole of traditional acupuncture (those parts that are valid, anyway) can be reinterpreted in terms of trigger points. Since the notion of trigger points is itself not widely understood within Western medicine, we need to spend a few moments in clarifying it. So, what are trigger points?

For the moment, we may define a trigger point as a tender area, often in muscle, from which pain may radiate to distant areas in the body. There is much more to say about the idea than this and I return to it in more detail in the next chapter, but this definition will do for the moment.

Brief history of the origin of the trigger point idea

Textbooks of medicine published in the first half of the twentieth century contained vague allusions to disorders called 'fibrositis' and 'muscular rheumatism' but the nature of these was quite unclear. However, important experiments had already been carried out, especially by J.H. Kellgren at London's University Hospital Medical School in the late

1930s. He noted that, in normal people, pain induced by stimulating muscles experimentally, for example by injecting hypertonic saline, was always diffuse and was often referred to other areas.

Kellgren also looked at patients suffering from 'fibrositis'. He found that they often had extremely tender areas in their muscles and also areas of referred pain, which were not generally tender. Injection of the tender areas with local anaesthetic often alleviated the patients' symptoms.

In other experiments, Kellgren and others discovered that if deep structures such as interspinous ligaments, tendons, joints, and periosteum were stimulated, there was extensive radiation of pain. The radiation patterns were constant and, Kellgren claimed, corresponded to areas of segmental innervation, which he called sclerotomes by analogy with dermatomes and myotomes. However, later investigators did not agree that referral from these deep structures followed simple segmental patterns.

An orthopaedic surgeon, A. Steindler, seems to have been the first to refer to 'trigger points'. It was however another American physician, Janet Travell, who popularized the term, beginning in the 1940s. Travell described what she called myofascial pain syndromes in relation to trigger points. Each muscle, she claimed, has its own characteristic pattern of pain referral, so a given type of pain may be related to a trigger point in a particular muscle. She continued to work on this over the years, and in the 1980s, in conjunction with her colleague David Simons, produced the first authoritative textbook on the subject. These authors described numerous trigger points and explained the method of inactivating them, which was mainly stretching after spraying the affected muscle with a cooling spray in order to relax it; but they also used injections of local anaesthetic, which is of course quite similar to acupuncture.

Trigger points and acupuncture

When Western doctors began to take acupuncture seriously in the 1970s and 1980s, they noticed resemblances between acupuncture points and trigger points. It was found that practically all the trigger points described in the Western literature had a classic acupuncture point close to them, and, conversely, about 70 per cent of classic acupuncture points had a trigger point close to them. Moreover, the Chinese had long recognized the existence of *ah shi* (Oh yes!) points: that is, sites that were not classic acupuncture points but which might become tender in disease and which could be needled. It was only a small step from this to equating acupuncture with the treatment of trigger points.

Some modern acupuncturists now base their treatment entirely on needling trigger points. When approached in this way, acupuncture certainly sounds less alien than in its traditional version, although it still suffers from the disadvantage that doctors are not taught anything about trigger points in their ordinary medical training. A more serious disadvantage is that not all the effective needling sites are tender; but a non-tender site cannot be called a trigger point. Thus there must be more to acupuncture than trigger points.

Mann's 'new concept' acupuncture (Mann, 2000)

In his book *Reinventing Acupuncture: a new concept of ancient medicine*, Felix Mann has put forward a view of acupuncture with which mine has a good deal in common. He disbelieves in the existence of 'points' and 'meridians' as commonly understood, and he thinks that trigger points, though important, are not the whole story. He notes that, in some patients, a needle inserted anywhere in the body will have some effect; the question that then arises is how to narrow the field down so as to give more precise recommendations for treating different types of symptoms. Here he uses two main guides.

One is the characteristic pattern of radiation from various needling sites. He finds, for example, that if one needles the periosteum in the sacroiliac joint region, a sensation, whose character is often difficult to describe, frequently travels down the lower limb, but the distance to which it goes, and the path taken, are widely variable from patient to patient. Similar patterns may occur when other sites are needled, and give, he claims, an important indication for deciding where to insert the needles. The other guide, to which he also attaches considerable importance, is local tenderness. However, he notes that a site on the dorsum of the foot (LR3), which he is particularly fond of using, is often not tender. He finds that effective needling sites are very variable in size; in some people they may be large.

In summary, then, Mann's version of acupuncture is similar in a number of respects to trigger point acupuncture but is wider in scope. He rejects almost all of traditional acupuncture and has substituted his own terminology for that of the traditional system, so that, for example, instead of referring to GB20 he speaks of the trapezius/occiput area. In addition to revising the terminology he has made several other distinctive contributions to modern acupuncture: these include the use of periosteal needling (not found in the traditional system), the recognition of the class of 'strong reactors' (again, not found in the traditional system), and the use of very brief gentle stimulation ('micro-acupuncture'). All of these have done much to make acupuncture both effective and quick to perform, and his view of acupuncture brought about a radical rationalization of acupuncture for many doctors, including me, in the 1970s.

Can we find common ground among the various approaches?

If we look at the four 'modernist' approaches to point selection summarized above, we see that there is a fair amount of common ground among them. For example, the segmental theme reappears in Gunn's radiculopathy, as does the idea of trigger points. There is also common ground with the traditional system, for at least some of the traditional acupuncture points could be reinterpreted as trigger points. Mann, likewise, includes trigger points and segmental needling by implication. My conclusion is that all these modernist ways of describing where to needle are valid but each has certain limitations if taken too literally. I find Mann's the most congenial of the four. Like him, I attach considerable importance to radiation. Local tenderness is, I think, also important, but perhaps less so than radiation. Neither tenderness nor radiation, however, is an infallible guide to where to insert the needles. This is particularly true for periosteal acupuncture. I use this extensively for treating joints, and often there are local tender areas to be found around the joints. I am not convinced, however, that it is necessary to needle these selectively; anywhere in the region of the joint seems to be equally effective.

The perhaps rather unwelcome fact is that, for some sites that are effective, there is no real guide other than experience; they just seem to work in practice and at present there isn't much more that one can say about them. There must presumably be some neurophysiological explanation for their effectiveness, but we shall have to wait for an explanation until we know more.

What I should like to do here is to amalgamate all the foregoing views in order to construct a comprehensive modern description of choosing where to needle. This method, I believe, makes room for certain facts and observations that are otherwise difficult to accommodate, and also avoids the ever-present temptation to theorize too freely.

The temptation to theorize prematurely

It seems to me that a great deal of what is written about acupuncture from the practical standpoint is prematurely attached to theory. Practitioners of modern acupuncture have an understandable wish to provide a pathophysiological basis for their treatments that will make them appear rational to critics, but this can lead them to put forward rather shaky arguments at times. Gunn's radiculopathy theory has some shortcomings in this respect, and another example is provided by the 'piriformis syndrome', which has been well reviewed by Cummings (2000) (see also Chapter 12). Earlier authors often stated or implied that this disorder was due to entrapment of all or part of the sciatic nerve by the piriformis muscle, but it can apparently also arise from trigger points in this muscle, without any entrapment. Cummings therefore defines it as 'a pain syndrome derived from the piriformis muscle, with or without sciatic nerve entrapment'. He mentions that other nerves may also be entrapped, particularly the superior and inferior gluteal nerves.

Cummings is surely right to avoid particularizing the diagnosis to include entrapment, but this raises the question: how useful is the label anyway? What is so special about the piriformis? Why not a gluteus medius syndrome or a gluteus minimus syndrome, since trigger points in these muscles may also give rise to referred pain in the buttock or leg? One could multiply this to postulate as many syndromes as there are muscles in the body, but I am not sure that it adds much to our understanding, and the danger of using a term like 'piriformis syndrome' is that it may suggest to the reader a degree of certainty about the pathological anatomy that is not justified. The presence of sciatic nerve entrapment is hardly ever verified in patients with the relevant symptoms, nor do we know how common it is for 'entrapment' to be present without causing symptoms.

We need to remember that medical diagnosis isn't an exact science. Postmortems are carried out much less frequently now than a few decades ago, but when they are done they suggest that diagnoses made in life are often mistaken; serious discrepancies between antemortem and postmortem diagnosis are found in 30–34 per cent of cases (During & Cation, 2000; Harris & Blundell, 1991; Hjorth *et al.*, 1994; Rao & Rangwala, 1990). Even with the aid of sophisticated modern diagnostic techniques, therefore, we are often misled about what is happening inside the bodies of our patients, and such investigations are often not used in patients receiving acupuncture. The fact is that, at present, it's difficult to explain many of the phenomena of acupuncture. I therefore prefer to keep my thinking on the purely descriptive level. There are clinical observations that are currently difficult to explain theoretically but which can certainly be made by anyone who cares to do so. Here are some of them.

● In some people, and for some disorders, it makes comparatively little difference where the needles are placed.
● There appears to be a 'generalized stimulation' effect, whereby a patient's sense of wellbeing can be improved and various disorders influenced by needling. Like diffuse noxious inhibitory control, this can be non-specific; it can result from inserting a needle almost anywhere, although certain sites, e.g. LR3, seem to be especially effective in this respect.
● In other cases needling needs to be more or less specific, but the area of effective needling is very variable; it may be quite large (i.e. several centimetres in diameter or even more). Trigger point acupuncture is sometimes of this nature, although at other times it seems to be necessary to needle the trigger point very accurately.
● It is sometimes possible to get a strong therapeutic effect from sites which are not noticeably tender to pressure. It is therefore incorrect to say that acupuncture is synonymous with the treatment of trigger points.

- Periosteal needling (possibly a form of sclerotomal segmental acupuncture) is effective for joint problems.
- Needling or otherwise stimulating certain areas of the body will characteristically give rise to radiation to other areas. This phenomenon can be used therapeutically to influence disorders in those secondary areas.
- Minimalist acupuncture ('micro-acupuncture' – Mann) is surprisingly effective in some patients and indeed is at times more effective than 'standard' acupuncture.

New terminology: the 'acupuncture treatment area'
(Campbell, 1999)

On the basis of these observations I have introduced a new term. I apologise for this, since I don't think we want more jargon than is absolutely necessary, but none of the existing vocabulary expresses what I have in mind. I have therefore coined the term 'acupuncture treatment area' (ATA) to refer to possible sites of needle insertion.

An ATA may be defined as a site anywhere in the body at which needles may be inserted to produce a therapeutic effect, either locally or at a distance.

ATAs may be of any size, which is one reason for using 'area' rather than 'point' to name them. Some are quite small, perhaps a centimetre or less in diameter, while others are much larger; indeed, the phenomenon of diffuse noxious inhibitory control (DNIC) described in Chapter 3 means that the whole body can be thought of as an ATA, since DNIC is, by definition, not confined to any single site.

The depth of ATAs is also variable. Some are deep within muscles or at the level of the periosteum, while others are near the surface (to explain the effectiveness of micro-acupuncture). ATAs must always be thought of three-dimensionally.

ATAs and trigger points

The distinction between ATAs and trigger points is important. A trigger point, by definition, is at least moderately tender. An ATA may be tender but need not be. Thus, all trigger points are ATAs, but not all ATAs are trigger points.

Some examples of ATAs

- A locally painful area may itself be an ATA; this is the simplest kind that exists. The *ah shi* points described in the traditional system are of this kind. Some people object that needling the painful site itself isn't proper acupuncture, but this seems to me to be absurd; anyway, for those who want to find authority for the practice, there are classical texts going back as far as the seventh century CE which describe it (Needham & Gwei-Djen, 1980).

● Classic acupuncture points, if they exist, will be ATAs.
● Sites of generalized stimulation: certain sites, such as LR3 and probably LI4, are classic acupuncture points but, I suggest, are best regarded as ATAs from which it is possible to produce a strong generalized effect.
● The piriformis muscle is an example of an ATA; symptoms could arise from this muscle either because of sciatic nerve entrapment or because of trigger points, and it's impossible to tell which by means of clinical examination.
● The periosteum around a joint is a (fairly poorly localized) ATA.
● For people who accept the validity of auriculotherapy, the outer ear is an ATA, which contains numerous mini-ATAs inside it.
● As noted above, the whole body can be thought of as a kind of macro-ATA, since diffuse noxious inhibitory control is a generalized response from anywhere in the body.

Advantages of the ATA concept

I would claim that introducing the ATA concept has a number of advantages.

● It avoids the danger of getting tied prematurely to any particular theoretical framework, which may need to be modified or superseded as research in acupuncture advances.
● It allows for the introduction of new methods of treatment, since these are not obliged to conform to theoretical expectations.
● I think it is a true reflection of what most modernist acupuncture practitioners are actually doing, because they are generally more flexible in their practice than in their theory. Informal conversations with experienced acupuncturists seem to confirm this view.

The last point seems to me to be particularly important. When one starts out in acupuncture it is quite difficult to avoid thinking of it as a very esoteric subject, and this view is sometimes reinforced by teachers. This isn't true. Acupuncture itself is relatively simple, given a good knowledge of anatomy. What's difficult is knowing when to apply it. Provided you have a certain minimum level of manual dexterity, your success rate in acupuncture will be approximately in proportion to your general clinical success rate. If you are getting good results with your existing treatments, especially manual treatments, you will get good results with acupuncture. Acupuncture is of a piece with the rest of clinical practice.

Beginners may get the impression that there is a firmly established body of rather arcane knowledge which must be gradually acquired, so that becoming an expert acupuncturist is largely a matter of learning more and more acupuncture points with their specific properties and effects. As time goes by, however, the aspiring acupuncturist is likely to find that this rather simplistic view of the matter doesn't correspond to what actually obtains. Different teachers of acupuncture have quite divergent ideas about how to choose which points to needle, as well as about the duration and intensity of needling and other matters. This can create a certain amount of confusion in students' minds. The remedy, I suggest, is to understand the basic principles and then to apply them without too many preconceptions.

There is a commonly held view about acupuncture which goes something like this. There are hundreds of acupuncture points, which all have specific effects that must be learned; improving your skill depends on learning more and more points, and the more points you know, the better your results will be. If you believe this, acupuncture is inevitably going to appear complex, requiring years of study in order to become expert at it. Experienced acupuncturists, if caught in unguarded moments, will often admit that this isn't really true; I certainly don't believe it myself. I think that precision of needling is often, though not always, relatively unimportant. On the other hand, we shouldn't go to the opposite extreme and say that it makes no difference at all where the needles are placed. So how do we go about choosing where to needle?

First, we recognize that there are certain sites (ATAs) from which radiation of sensations is normally propagated in particular patterns. Needling the ATAs in question can then treat symptoms in the relevant areas. However, we also remember that the patterns described are only averages; individual patients may and do present with different radiation patterns, so it's important to remain flexible in our thinking. Descriptions of ATAs are guides, not invariable rules; skeleton keys to try in the symptom lock. And new ones will be discovered from time to time; probably every experienced acupuncturist has found some needling sites that have not yet been described in books.

Next, we think about the history and pathology, because these will often give a clue to where to try inserting the needles. For example, I have found an ATA at the back of the thigh which is also a trigger zone and may be activated by sitting on a hard chair which presses on the hamstrings; it refers pain to the front of the thigh above the knee. I haven't seen this described anywhere (though of course it may be).

Finally, if all else fails, and we still want to try acupuncture, we can use generalized stimulation, which in practice means needling the hands or feet, but especially the feet.

The ATA approach to acupuncture is deliberately not overprescriptive. It is meant for people who don't necessarily want to be presented with a book of rules to follow blindly but who like to try to understand what they are doing and are prepared to think for themselves. In the traditional system enormous importance is generally attached to locating acupuncture points exactly, and the rather 'free-style' approach to acupuncture I advocate may appear unsettling to some. Newcomers sometimes yearn for firm instructions: they want to be told that in disorder A you should put the needles in points x, y, and z, while in disorder B you should put them in points p, q, and r, and that provided you do this you should get the hoped-for results. But things are not so simple, and confident instructions of this kind really do students a disservice. (Please understand that this applies to postgraduates, who are, or should be, used to thinking critically for themselves; the position might be different if one were teaching acupuncture to undergraduates.)

ATA terminology: recording the treatment

How are ATAs to be named? Some writers, e.g. Mann and Gunn, avoid using acupuncture terminology altogether, but the difficulty with this is that one may become involved in clumsy circumlocutions. I therefore favour an admittedly inconsistent approach. When an ATA happens to coincide with a standard acupuncture point I use that name. Thus I refer to LR3, GB21 and so on, even though I don't think one needs to needle these sites with the precision that the traditionalists insist on. Other sites don't correspond to traditional points and then I sometimes use anatomical terminology (gluteus medius site, sacroiliac joint, greater trochanter of femur, etc.). I have also invented a few names for ATAs, as will appear in Part 3; however, I have been sparing with these neologisms and only use them when it is more or less unavoidable.

These principles form the basis of recording the treatment using ATA terminology. It is obviously essential to do this adequately, both for clinical purposes and because of medicolegal considerations. Some people advocate marking the sites on charts, and this is certainly an option if the charts are available; however, even so I think it is desirable to supplement the pictorial depiction with a verbal description.

As well as the site needled, I record the side (L or R), and in some cases the depth, although I generally do this only if it is in some way exceptional: either deep (periosteal) or superficial (minimalist or micro-acupuncture). Similarly, a moderate amount of manual stimulation is assumed: if none is done or (very rarely) strong stimulation is used I record that.

It is also important to record any immediate effects, such as an increase in the range of movement, and it is certainly essential to note any adverse effects such as fainting or other unusual phenomena. It is useful, although not essential, to use a visual analogue scale (VAS) to record the intensity of the symptoms.

Two examples follow.

(Comments are given in parentheses.)

Mrs B

(A 47-year-old woman who has had pain in the right side of her neck for three months. She is otherwise well.)

First visit
Complaint: pain in right side of neck (symptomatic description only; the cause of most back and neck pain is unknown and we should acknowledge this).

   Finding on examination: rotation to R reduced to 45 degrees
   VAS = 6 (visual analogue scale – not essential)
   TP ++ (moderately active trigger) at the level of C3 R

Treatment: GB21, GB20.5 LR; also above-mentioned TP (two classic acupuncture points on each side; also a trigger not corresponding to a classic point. See Part 3 for locations of these points.)
Effects: Faint! (Important to record this for future reference.)

Second visit
Result of first treatment: Initial aggravation; now better.

   VAS = 3. Finding on examination: Neck rotation = 60 degrees (improved).
   Feeling better in herself
   Fewer headaches

Treatment: Repeat needling, more lightly (in view of fainting previously).

Mr F

(A 60-year-old man, suffering for sciatica for some time.)

First visit
Complaint: Sciatica 6 months.

   Clinical findings: Lumbar spasm
   Straight leg raising 50 degrees L, 80 degrees R. Tenderness of spine of L5. Gluteal TP +++ in R gluteal region (anatomical description of location of TP)
   VAS = 6

Treatment: L5 periosteally (note depth). SIJ L (sacroiliac joint; standard ATA term). Gluteal TP: radiation down leg reproduces pain (important clinical fact).

Second visit
Result: Dramatically better for two days; now relapsing.

   Sleeping better than for many weeks.
   VAS = 3

Treatment: Repeat acupuncture as above.

The above features are recorded at every treatment. At follow-up one should also note the outcome of the previous treatment, with particular attention being paid to the way in which the symptoms evolved in the first few days. Was there an aggravation? If so, how long did it last? How severe was it? Was it followed by an improvement? How long did any improvement last? Have any new symptoms developed since the previous treatment?

The patient is re-examined physically at each attendance and changes in the number, tenderness, or distribution of trigger points are noted, as well as changes in the range of movement. The patient's general state should also be considered, since changes in mood, sometimes long-lasting, can follow acupuncture.

Because acupuncture terminology is not standardized (at least, if one is not following the traditional system), it's important to reach agreement on the descriptive system to be used within a unit, if more than one therapist is practising acupuncture. Even if you are working on your own, it's essential, if only for medicolegal reasons, to have a standardized method of recording your treatment that could, if necessary, be explained clearly to someone else.

References

Baldry P.E. (1998) *Acupuncture, Trigger Points, and Musculoskeletal Pain.* Churchill Livingstone, Edinburgh.

Bekkering R. & van Bussel R. (1998) Segmental acupuncture. In: *Medical Acupuncture: a Western scientific approach* (eds Filshie J. & White A). Churchill Livingstone, Edinburgh.

Campbell A. (1999). Acupuncture: where to place the needles and for how long. *Acupuncture in Medicine*, 17; 113–17.

Cummings M. (2000). Piriformis syndrome. *Acupuncture in Medicine*, 17; 108–21.

During S. & Cation L. (2000) The educational value of autopsy in a residency training program. *Archives of Internal Medicine*, 160; 997–9.

Gunn C.C. (1998) Acupuncture and the peripheral nervous system. In: *Medical Acupuncture: a Western scientific approach* (eds Filshie J. & White A.). Churchill Livingstone, Edinburgh.

Harris M.D. & Blundell J.W. (1991) Audit of necropsies in a British general hospital. *Journal of Clinical Pathology*, 44; 862–5.

Hjorth L. *et al.* (1994) Importance of the autopsy rate. A comparison between clinical assessment and findings at autopsies during the periods: 1 July 1980–30 June 1981 and 1 July 1990–30 June 1991. *Ugeschrift for Laeger*, 156; 4459–61.

Mann F. (2000) *Reinventing Acupuncture: a new concept of ancient medicine* (second edition). Butterworth-Heinemann, London.

Needham J. & Gwei-Djen L. (1980) *Celestial Lancets: a history of acupuncture and moxa.* Cambridge University Press, Cambridge.

Rao M.G. & Rangwala A.F. (1990) Diagnostic yield from 231 autopsies in a community hospital. *American Journal of Clinical Pathology*, 93; 486–90.

Chapter 7

The ATA concept in practice

Having described what I mean by an ATA, I am now ready to explain how I go about using acupuncture in practice. We can summarize the approach as follows. There are four basic principles in the kind of acupuncture I use.

1. Most disorders amenable to acupuncture are treated by needling either the affected area itself or a relevant ATA at some distance away from it. These ATAs may or may not be tender (may or may not be trigger points).
2. Some disorders are best treated by generalized stimulation, and this can always be used as an adjunct to the previous form of needling.
3. Intrinsic joint disease is usually treated by periosteal needling in the neighbourhood of the affected joint.
4. Getting the amount of stimulation right is crucial. Usually this means doing less rather than more.

For me, pretty much the whole of acupuncture consists in applying these four principles in different combinations. Some amplification is however needed, particularly concerning the use of trigger points.

The relevance of trigger points to acupuncture

As we saw in the last chapter, there is a widespread tendency among Western acupuncturists to describe what they do almost entirely in terms of deactivating trigger points (Baldry, 1998). On this view of the matter, whatever is valuable in the traditional system can be preserved in the form of trigger point acupuncture. Now, trigger points are certainly important, but they aren't the universal answer. Circular arguments enter into the story rather easily here; even Travell and Simons are not immune. For example, they describe what they call trigger points in the abdominal wall, which they think are responsible for chronic diarrhoea, and in the interosseus muscles of the hand, which they say are associated with osteoarthritis and Heberden's nodes (Travell & Simons, 1983). I agree with these associations, but the sites in question are by no means invariably tender. They therefore shouldn't be called trigger points, which are tender by definition. They are, however, ATAs, since they can be used therapeutically.

Periosteal needling, in particular, doesn't need to be done at sites of tenderness. Tender sites may be present near joints, and are often advocated for treatment. Needling them certainly works, but so does needling non-tender sites in the same region, and I'm not convinced that there is much difference between the two methods.

In spite of these criticisms, however, I do recognize and use trigger points in muscles and ligaments extensively and, if they are present, the chances of success are probably increased. In view of this, we need to review the trigger point concept at this point in more detail and to expand on the rather sketchy outline given in the last chapter.

The characteristics of trigger points
(Travell & Simons, 1983; 1992)

Trigger points may be found in muscles, tendons, ligaments, and joint capsules. They are classified as either latent or active. Latent trigger points can be found in normal people, in whom they give rise to no symptoms. For example, the midpoint of the trapezius muscle is a latent trigger point, and so is the infraglenoid tubercle, on the scapula below the glenoid cavity just above the origin of the long head of the triceps. Firm pressure on these and similar sites is painful in almost everyone. An active trigger point is one from which pain is felt spontaneously, either locally or at some distance from it, in the zone of referred pain. Some active trigger points develop from pre-existing latent triggers, but others arise at sites that were not previously tender at all.

In spite of a fair amount of research and quite a lot of speculation, there is no general agreement about what trigger points are. Those that are in muscles possess increased electrical activity, which can be demonstrated if an insulated needle with just the tip exposed is inserted into them, but they show no definite or constant histological features (A. Ward, personal communication). It is possible that they are maintained centrally, by activity originating from the spinal cord. A noxious stimulus could cause reflex maintenance of nociceptor activity in the periphery via an outflow through the sympathetic system; another suggestion is that the trauma may cause reflex maintenance of muscle spasm via motoneurons.

Once they have arisen or become active, trigger points may persist and cause symptoms for long periods: weeks, months, or even years. On the other hand, they can often also be abolished, at least temporarily, by simple pressure as well as by the insertion of a needle or in other ways. Lack of awareness about the length of time a trigger point may remain active after an injury has often led doctors to suspect a psychosomatic disorder or even malingering in patients with persistent pain, yet often a complete and permanent cure can be achieved in such cases by the insertion of a simple acupuncture needle.

Trigger points can become active in a number of ways. Trauma, sudden strain, or excessive use of the muscle may do this; so, too, may continued overuse or prolonged contraction, as may occur in people who are psychologically tense. Emotional factors are certainly concerned in their genesis and maintenance. Other causes include prolonged immobilization and infections; and sometimes the cause is unknown.

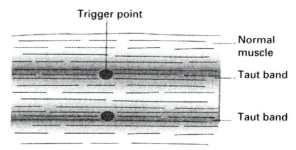

Muscle with taut bands and trigger points (plan view)

Travell and Simons distinguish between primary and satellite trigger points; the satellites develop in areas of referred pain. For example, patients with sciatica may have a primary trigger point in the gluteal region and a number of satellite trigger points in the limb below. The term 'secondary trigger point' refers to trigger points that may develop in antagonist or synergist muscles.

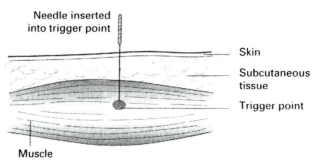

Muscle with trigger point – insertion of needle

An important feature of trigger points is that they may be associated with taut bands in the muscles. These are thought to be zones of increased contractility. Like trigger points, they may come and go with surprising rapidity.

Examining patients for trigger points

The art of examining patients for trigger points requires practice to learn. It is not taught to medical students so doctors coming to acupuncture have to acquire it. There are two basic techniques. For flat muscles, such as the gluteal muscles, the skin and subcutaneous tissues are moved transversely across the line of the muscle fibres. Travell and Simons describe the action as like that of feeling corduroy. A way of simulating it to some extent is to lay a few pencils side by side on a table, cover them with a cloth, and then move the cloth with the finger across the pencils so that they roll beneath it. The middle finger seems to be more sensitive than the index finger for the purpose, and I find that my left hand is more sensitive than my right, but this may be an individual peculiarity.

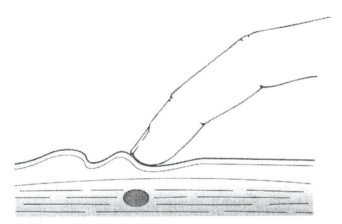

Palpating trigger point

The alternative technique of examination, which is required for strap muscles such as the sternomastoid and also for areas such as the anterior and posterior axillary folds, is to use a pincer action, gripping the muscle between thumb and middle finger and drawing the skin and subcutaneous tissues across the underlying muscle as if trying to pull them off it.

It is important to have the muscles under slight tension, though not too much, when searching for trigger points. A totally relaxed muscle cannot be examined in this way, nor can a firmly contracted one.

No instruments are required for detecting trigger points; you need only your fingers. It takes time, however, to build up an awareness of how much pressure to apply. We start with fairly gentle pressure, both to avoid causing unnecessary pain and because, in some patients, this is more effective; we then apply progressively firmer pressure in an attempt to elicit tenderness. In certain situations, such as the gluteal muscles, considerable pressure may need to be exerted, because the affected muscles, such as the piriformis, lie at depth below other layers of muscle. In all this process of examination we need to keep the anatomy in mind and constantly try to maintain a three-dimensional mental image of what we are feeling.

Some degree of tenderness is normal in muscles if they are pressed sufficiently firmly. The acupuncturist therefore needs to form a mental, or rather a kinaesthetic, image of how much tenderness is to be expected for a particular degree of pressure at a given site. This varies according to the type of patient. In general, women have more latent trigger points than men, so a degree of tenderness in the trapezius muscle that would be accepted as normal in a woman might be abnormal in a man. But it's not only the absolute degree of tenderness that we need to be aware of; we also compare the two sides of the body, and differences here are particularly significant.

With practice, different degrees of tension can be felt in the muscles, and the above-mentioned strands of taut muscle can be identified; one particularly tender area in each of these strands will be found and this is the trigger point. Sometimes a strand of muscle will twitch under the finger as it slides across the tense strand; this indicates the site of the trigger point. A twitch of this kind can be elicited in most people in that portion of extensor digitorum that controls the middle finger. Another indication is the so-called 'jump sign'; 'flinch sign' might be more accurate because the patient pulls sharply away as the trigger point is encountered. And, of course, patients will generally tell you that they experience pain as the trigger point is pressed.

The locations of trigger points in the various muscles are described in textbooks. As a general rule, referral of pain is from axis to periphery and from proximal to distal, so this gives an idea of where one should be looking for trigger points. However, every patient is different and there is no substitute for careful clinical examination without preconceptions. Restriction of individual movements also gives clues; for example, if a patient has restricted neck rotation this would suggest the presence of trigger points in the opposite sternomastoid since this muscle is responsible for rotation (although other muscles in the neck could of course be affected as well).

Fibromyalgia versus myofascial pain

Up to this point we have been looking at trigger points in the context of what Travell and Simons call the myofascial pain syndrome. That is, we have been talking about fairly localized tender areas and radiation of pain therefrom. However, there are patients who have some of the features of myofascial pain but who seem to suffer from a different disorder, which is nowadays often labelled fibromyalgia. The main differences are as follows.

● Fibromyalgia affects women much more than men.
● Pain is widespread in fibromyalgia, whereas in myofascial pain it is usually localized although more than one area of the body may affected.
● Patients with fibromyalgia often wake up feeling tired. Sleep may also be disturbed in myofascial pain because of the pain, but sleep disturbance is not part of the syndrome as such.
● Patients with fibromyalgia often have morning stiffness and fatigue.
● Antidepressants may help patients with fibromyalgia, although this is not necessarily because they are depressed. (However, emotional upsets and stress do seem to be related to the onset of fibromyalgia.) Antidepressants don't help myofascial pain. Neither fibromyalgia nor myofascial pain respond to non-steroidal anti-inflammatory drugs (NSAIDs).
● Fibromyalgia appears to be part of a spectrum of related disorders, including irritable bowel syndrome, tension headaches, and primary dysmenorrhoea. This is not true of myofascial pain.
● The prognosis of the two disorders differs. Myofascial pain generally responds well to acupuncture whereas fibromyalgia does not; at best, acupuncture seems to give partial relief for a short time in fibromyalgia, perhaps for two or three weeks. This can present the acupuncturist with a difficult problem in the case of patients who find even this brief remission worth while, since the disorder can last for many months or even years; in fact, indefinitely.

Acupuncture and the deactivation of trigger points

Acupuncture is simply one method among others for deactivating trigger points. Other methods including simple pressure ('acupressure'), 'stretch and spray' as used by Travell and Simons, and the injection of various substances (local anaesthetic, corticosteroids) into the site. (It seems likely that at least some of the effectiveness of corticosteroid injection is due to the irritant effect of the injection rather than to its anti-inflammatory effect.) In fact, it's very possible that other forms of manual therapy, including some physiotherapy techniques, manipulation as used by osteopaths and chiropractors, and plain massage, all act in much the same way. There is therefore nothing magical about the use of an acupuncture needle. However, this form of therapy has certain advantages. It is more effective and long-lasting than simple manual pressure. Although the response to a corticosteroid injection may sometimes be more long-lasting than the response to acupuncture, such injections cannot be repeated more than a few times because of unwanted effects, whereas acupuncture can be performed as many times as necessary.

Acupuncture for trigger point disorders, then, consists in the insertion of needles (some people prefer to call this 'dry needling' or 'intramuscular stimulation' – Gunn.) But this can be done in a number of ways, and as usual there is no firm guidance to help us choose the best. The following questions arise.

1. Is it desirable to try to direct the needle right into the trigger point or is it enough just to needle the subcutaneous tissues over the site of the trigger point, without entering it? (This is more or less what I referred to earlier as minimalist acupuncture.)
2. If there are quite numerous trigger points, should we treat all of them at each sitting or just the most tender ones?

It can be very difficult to make up one's mind firmly about such questions in acupuncture. Opinions may be formed on perhaps inadequate evidence, and thereafter you may dig yourself deeper and deeper into the same trench. This is a general problem affecting all forms of therapy, such as acupuncture, where there is little firm research evidence to guide one. Suppose you are using a particular treatment method which seems to work in a reasonable proportion of cases. There is little incentive to try an alternative method instead, and indeed it might seem rather questionable from the ethical standpoint to do so, since if a given treatment appears to be helping a patient, do you have the right to try something else which might not be so good? Of course, you could legitimately try an alternative on the next patient you saw, but the difficulty with this is that there are so many variables in acupuncture that it would be difficult to assess the reasons for any difference that might emerge.

Decisions about such matters therefore have to be based largely on experience, but this isn't a wholly trustworthy guide. Experience is a good thing, no doubt, but it needs to be kept constantly under critical review, otherwise it can all too easily result simply in confirming ourselves in our own prejudices. What we need is good objective evidence, but this is hard to come by in acupuncture. Once again, we hear the usual refrain: more trials, please. But trials will take a long time to carry out and may not give a clear-cut answer even when they are done, and meanwhile there are patients to see and we have make up our minds about what to do.

With regard to the first question, my own impression, for what it's worth, is that sometimes it makes a difference if you insert the needle right into the trigger point and sometimes it doesn't. In treating myself, which is one way of refining one's technique by watching what happens after needling, I have found that it is sometimes essential to get the needle accurately into the trigger point. And, as a rule, when I am treating patients I like to needle the trigger points as precisely as possible, with the usual accompaniment of de qi. In such cases I feel that I have achieved something, and the results are often good. However, I also see good results after treatments in which I have not done this, so I am quite prepared to believe that there are at least some cases in which it isn't essential. Superficial needling is certainly more comfortable for the patient, and there seem to be some people in whom it is more effective than deep needling (compare Mann's preference for 'micro-acupuncture'). Deciding how much stimulation to give in a particular patient is, I believe, one of the most critical judgements in acupuncture, and in so far as 'advanced' acupuncture may be said to exist, this is what it mainly consists in. (The other part is good selection of patients and symptoms to treat.)

I therefore generally try to visualize where and at what depth the trigger point lies, and then aim for it. Different sensations can be felt as the needle advances. The most characteristic is a grating or 'creaking' sensation as the trigger point is encountered; the needle may also be gripped very firmly, particularly in the gluteal region, as soon as any stimulation is given. Sometimes the trigger point may be hard to locate with the needle, and in that case stronger stimulation may be required, but this is unusual; as a rule, if the needle is partially withdrawn, re-angled, and advanced again, the trigger point will be found. At times, indeed, the needle may then be locked in the trigger point, and it's necessary to wait a few minutes before withdrawing it.

One practical difficulty that may arise when performing acupuncture in this way is that the trigger point may be inactivated temporarily simply by the examination used to locate it. You palpate the muscle, find a trigger point you want to treat, and go away for a minute to fetch a needle. When you return to the patient you can no longer find the trigger point, no matter how hard you press. To avoid this difficulty you can mark the site to be needled, using a skin pencil, but be careful not to make a cross and go through it, or you will tattoo the patient; rather, draw a circle round the tender area. In fact, I don't find it necessary to mark the spot in this way; with practice you can learn to mentally 'photograph' the site so that you remember where the trigger was. There are often small skin blemishes that will help you to do this.

The second question (about the number of triggers that should be treated on each occasion) is equally difficult to answer. We quite often read opinions stating firmly that all the triggers should be treated, otherwise the patient will not be helped. In my experience this isn't true, and I think that by doing this one risks causing bad aggravations. My own preference is to do as little as possible, especially on the first occasion. I usually treat two or three sites, not more, and sometimes only one. When I have treated these sites and obtained perhaps a 50 per cent improvement in range of movement, I generally leave it at that. Quit while you're ahead. When I have yielded to the temptation to continue and try to get a further improvement, I have sometimes undone the good I had initially achieved. Doing less therefore seems to be better than doing more. When the patient returns a week or two later I often find that the original trigger points have disappeared but that new ones have arisen; it is as if one were progressively uncovering different layers of trigger activity. I have also found that needling sites of referred pain, for example in the leg in patients with sciatica or at the insertion of the deltoid muscle in the arm in patients with pain referred from the neck, is ineffective or can even make matters worse. But others have had different experiences.

These are just two of the very basic questions about acupuncture that are still unresolved. In the absence of firm guidelines from research we have to trust to our own experience or the opinions of others whose judgement we respect, but we should always keep in mind the possibility that we may be wrong.

Trigger points versus ATAs: the trigger point concept in practice

As will by now have become clear, I attach a lot of importance to trigger points, but I don't think they are all-important. So, in practice, if you follow the method I'm suggesting, your thought processes go something like this. (Here I imagine that we are jointly interviewing a patient for the first time, keeping the possibility of using acupuncture in mind; which, if you are an acupuncture practitioner, will generally be the case, especially if the main complaint is one of pain.)

The first question is whether acupuncture is at all likely to be of use in this instance. The decision to try acupuncture will be based on patient characteristics as well as on the local pain features. The features mentioned in Chapter 5 as suggesting that someone may be a strong reactor are important, although the 'pseudo-strong reactor' category must also be kept in mind. Belief in acupuncture is irrelevant but fear is certainly important, since if someone is 'afraid of needles' acupuncture is unlikely to work. After a time one begins to develop a 'feel' for the kind of patient who is likely to do well; this presumably depends on picking up subtle signals from voice, body language, and other characteristics that one may not always be fully conscious of.

Let us suppose that the patient in question here seems likely to be at least a reasonable prospect for acupuncture so far as general characteristics are concerned. Next, we ask ourselves whether the disorder is a musculoskeletal one. Often the answer to this is obvious, but sometimes it is not.

- An elderly patient complains of creeping or crawling sensations on top of the head. These often arise from trigger points in the neck, so it may

well be musculoskeletal, but this is not something that is obvious to a
therapist who isn't familiar with the phenomenon.

● A unilateral watering eye may be caused by a trigger point at the base
  of the skull (GB20).

In other words, quite a number of common symptoms may be trigger
point disorders in disguise. Experience is important here; someone who is
not familiar with this form of treatment may not think of the possibility
that trigger points are involved in such cases.

If we suspect a trigger point disorder, we obviously make a search for
tender areas. But what if there are none? Does this mean that we have to
dismiss the possibility of using acupuncture from consideration? No,
because, if we use the ATA concept, we don't necessarily expect to find
tenderness at the place we intend to insert the needles. We therefore
choose a needling site, which may be the painful area itself or may be a
remote site from which sensations typically radiate to the area of pain. For
example, if there is diffuse pain in the back of the thigh, we might needle
the sacroiliac region. In this case we are not using trigger point
acupuncture because no trigger point is actually present, but the treatment
is much the same as if a trigger point were present.

Perhaps we think that the disorder is not a trigger point one but rather
is due to damage to a particular joint, perhaps by osteoarthritis. In that
case we think of using periosteal acupuncture. Since this is a relatively
imprecise method we can simply choose a site to needle that is reasonably
accessible, because it is near the surface. Ideally, I like to needle both
sides of a joint but often it is enough to needle only one side. Just one
needle may be used, or two or three sites around the joint may be
stimulated. In the case of a joint, however, we need to keep the limits of
the joint capsule in mind; it's unnecessarily risky to insert acupuncture
needles into the joint itself in view of the (remote) possibility of causing
a joint infection.

Perhaps we don't think that the problem is musculoskeletal, but
nevertheless acupuncture seems worth considering. There could be
several reasons for this: the disorder might be one for which acupuncture
often gives good results, such as ulcerative colitis; the patient might be
keen to have acupuncture (and there is no reason not to try it); the disorder
is an obscure one, which several consultants have failed to find an
explanation for; or the patient is potentially a good acupuncture subject.
In all these cases we might try generalized stimulation, say at LR3.

Finally, the problem might be one that is unrelated to trigger points but
that often responds to needling a particular ATA. For example, trigeminal
neuralgia is often helped by needling the deep infratemporal fossa (as
described in Part 3).

I hope this outline of the thought processes that run through the mind
of a modern acupuncturist (this modern acupuncturist, anyway) will give
an indication of how this form of treatment can be applied in practice. The

techniques themselves are relatively simple; what matters is how, when, and how strongly they are applied.

To summarize, the questions one asks oneself are as follows:

- **Are these symptoms likely to respond to acupuncture?**
- **Is this patient likely to be a good or at least an average acupuncture responder?**
- **Is this likely to be a trigger point disorder?**
- **If no trigger points are present, are there ATAs that might work?**
- **Is there a chance that generalized stimulation might help?**

If the answers to any of these questions is yes, I would normally suggest acupuncture to the patient. This usually entails a reasonably detailed setting forth of what is going to happen and what the patient can expect to experience, because, as I explain in Part 4, it seems to be necessary to switch the patient's nervous system into 'treatment mode' before starting. (This has nothing to do with belief; it's simply a matter of acceptance of the therapeutic context.)

How much encouragement to give is a matter of individual judgement. My own practice is to tell the patient, as accurately as I can, what I think the chances of success will be. I generally include a warning that there is a failure rate of about 20–30 per cent in all acupuncture treatments, so if the patient happens to fall into the non-responder category the treatment won't work. Other practitioners like to use a great deal of positive reinforcement in order to maximize the placebo response and don't talk about possible failure rates, and this is quite legitimate. However, I prefer to be as objective as possible, presumably for temperamental reasons. My success rate, nevertheless, appears to be about the same as other people's, so perhaps the placebo effect is not as large in acupuncture as one might expect it to be.

References

Baldry P.E. (1998) *Acupuncture, trigger points and musculoskeletal pain.* Churchill Livingstone, Edinburgh.
Travell J.G. & Simons D.G. (1983) *Myofascial Pain and Dysfunction. The trigger point manual,* vol. 1. Williams & Wilkins, Baltimore.
Travell J.G. & Simons D.G. (1992) *Myofascial Pain and Dysfunction. The trigger point manual,* vol. 2. Williams & Wilkins, Baltimore.

Part 3

Chapter 8

Treatment: general introduction

Having read Part 2, you will no doubt be able to forecast the general approach to acupuncture that I shall use in this section of the book. I shall describe the various treatments that I've found to be successful, but I hope to do this without falling into the trap of writing a cookbook. When I describe a particular treatment, it is because I have found it to work, usually in a substantial number of cases, but that doesn't mean there are not alternatives that might work equally well. The treatments in question, in other words, are meant to be descriptive, not prescriptive. What I am seeking to convey is not a set of rules but rather a way of thinking about acupuncture. If I succeed in doing this I shall free you to adapt the principles of acupuncture to your own needs, and this is a great deal more useful than presenting you with rules. You will undoubtedly encounter clinical problems that have not come my way, but if you have grasped the general principle of acupuncture you may be able to devise treatments that apply in your particular circumstances and which may not have been recorded or even used before. Feel free to improvise.

This raises an important point about the accuracy of diagnosis. It cannot be said too emphatically that modern acupuncture is a method of treatment, not of diagnosis, and the general rule applies: diagnosis before treatment. The acupuncturist should therefore make every effort to reach a conventional anatomical and pathological diagnosis if at all possible. In fact, this is particularly important in the case of acupuncture, just because it can be an effective symptomatic treatment. The fact that a patient improves with acupuncture can never, by itself, be taken as showing that there is no serious pathology present. Diagnosis is needed both for prognosis and in order to exclude disorders that would be best treated in other ways.

However, in spite of best efforts, there will be many patients in whom, if one is honest, it is not possible to make a conventional diagnosis. It is often stated that in about 85 per cent of cases of backache the cause is unknown. It is false precision in such cases to claim a pathological accuracy that does not exist; it is misleading to say that a patient has spondylosis when the radiographs show simply the changes expected in a middle-aged individual. On the other hand, when the site of a problem can be identified anatomically, this will often suggest sites that it may be useful to needle.

A related question is, what may we reasonably expect acupuncture to achieve? We sometimes hear it stated or implied that it's possible to reverse pathology by needling people. If this is taken to mean, for example, that it can improve the radiographic appearances in osteoarthritis objectively, I have to say that there is no good evidence for this. Acupuncture can relieve pain in such disorders but that is all. The position is different where one is dealing with a disease that fluctuates in intensity, such as ulcerative colitis, which is capable of going into partial or even complete remission on its own. In such cases it is possible that acupuncture may move a patient into remission, and this indeed seems to happen sometimes in ulcerative colitis, although it would be misleading to speak of cure. In other cases (for example, migraine), there are no known pathological changes in between attacks, so the question of pathology reversal doesn't arise. In general, acupuncture should be thought of as a symptomatic treatment.

The descriptive method

The general approach I use in describing the treatments is regional. That is, I consider each region (head and neck, shoulder, upper limb and so on), listing the ATAs commonly found in each and the disorders that can be treated by needling them. This is a different arrangement from that found in medical textbooks, which go about things in a systemic way (cardiovascular system, digestive system, etc.). Quite a number of courses in modern acupuncture use the systemic approach, and when I started teaching acupuncture I did so myself. In particular, I made a separation between musculoskeletal and 'other' disorders. I then came to the conclusion that this was somewhat artificial and that it was better to follow a regional description. The chief reason for this is that the distinction between these two categories isn't always clear-cut.

For example, a site at the back of the skull corresponding to the classic acupuncture point GB20 can cause pain in the head, and can also cause watering of the eye on the affected side. Are we to call this a musculoskeletal symptom? It seems to be related to a musculoskeletal trigger point but it is not a pain. It often seems to be rather artificial to separate musculoskeletal and 'other' disorders.

Headaches are very frequently treated by acupuncturists who needle the neck, often with good results. It would be difficult to distinguish between headaches which are caused by musculoskeletal factors and those which are due to other causes. In other words, musculoskeletal and 'other' disorders overlap to a considerable extent and it is best to consider them all together.

Quite a number of patients present with symptoms that are not obviously musculoskeletal but which can be treated by needling trigger points. These could be thought of as musculoskeletal symptoms 'in disguise'; we shall encounter a number of examples as we go through the treatment of the various regions.

Types of spinal pain

It will become apparent as we go on that many of the symptoms to be described are either located in the spine or are referred from the spine to other parts of the body. The spine is a major focus of attention in acupuncture and we therefore need to summarize the main features of spinal pain at the outset; this description will set the stage for much of what follows.

It is helpful to distinguish three types of 'mechanical' spinal pain, as suggested by J.P. O'Brien (1984). All are likely to be made worse by movement, which distinguishes mechanical pain from pain due to inflammation or malignancy or referred to the spine from elsewhere. These more sinister varieties of pain are also likely to be worse at night or when the patient is supine. (See Chapter 12 for a summary of danger signs in back pain.)

Type A

Type A spinal pain is deep, dull, aching, and poorly localized. It may be felt in the back or may radiate to distant areas. The distribution of pain is fairly constant but it doesn't correspond with the known areas of supply of nerves or nerve roots. This 'sclerotome pain', as it has been called, may radiate to the eye, chest wall, elbow, groin, lower abdomen, or foot, and not surprisingly it can give rise to diagnostic problems. A great deal of acupuncture is concerned with the treatment of this kind of pain. All sorts of explanations have been advanced for type A pain but none is particularly convincing, and at present we have to say that the origin of this pain is unknown.

Type B

Type B pain is in a sense the reverse of type A pain. Instead of being diffuse and 'deep', it is felt at the site of trouble and is accurately localized. It arises from the superficial tissues (skin, fascia, superficial ligaments, tips of spinous processes, interspinous ligament). It generally responds well to acupuncture.

Type C

Type C pain is due to pressure on a nerve or nerve root. It takes the form of sharp 'electric shock' pain that shoots down a limb and typically has a dermatome distribution. There may be paralysis or weakness, loss of reflexes, paraesthesia or anaesthesia, or autonomic changes. Since this is due to direct pressure, it is not to be expected that needling trigger points or other sites would alleviate it, and acupuncture is indeed generally ineffective in this kind of pain. However, patients may have more than one kind of pain, so acupuncture may at least alleviate some of the symptoms if not all.

Reference

O'Brien J.P. (1984) In: *A Textbook of Pain* (eds Wall P.D. & Melzack R.). Churchill Livingstone, Edinburgh.

Chapter 9

The head and neck

This is one of the principal areas treated by acupuncturists. A wide range of disorders may cause pain in this region, including trauma (whiplash injury) and degenerative disease, although, as in other regions of the spine, the cause of pain often remains unknown. Whiplash injury is particularly troublesome; one prospective study found that 18 per cent of patients were still experiencing symptoms two years after the accident. The patients who continued to suffer in this way were older, were more likely to have had their heads in an inclined or rotated position at impact, had worse symptoms initially, and had more severe osteoarthritic changes on radiographic examination.

Herniation of cervical disks is another major cause of pain in the neck, shoulder, arm, and hand. It may be acute or subacute. Acute disk prolapse in young people is often due to trauma; in older patients the association with trauma is found less often and both disk disease and spondylosis may be present. Acupuncture cannot, of course, undo a disk prolapse, but, given the uncertainty about anatomical diagnosis in many cases of spinal pain, there is nothing to be lost by trying it a few times.

A man in his early 40s had severe neck pain, with radiation down his left arm. He was seen by a neurosurgeon who proposed to operate on his neck, although he warned the patient that it was possible that this would lead to quadriplegia if the operation was unsuccessful. Not surprisingly, the patient decided to explore the possibility of alternative treatment before agreeing to surgery. After two acupuncture treatments to his cervical articular column his pain was completely relieved and he did not require surgery.

Osteoarthritis of the cervical spine may cause pain that radiates into the back of the head, the shoulders, or the arms. It may cause paraesthesiae in the scalp, and may also cause headaches in the posterior occipital region via the C2–C4 nerve roots. Narrowing of the cervical spinal canal may compress the spinal cord and result in bladder symptoms as well as motor, sensory, and reflex changes in the legs; Lhermitte's sign (an electric-shock sensation elicited by neck flexion) may be present. Spinal cord compression doesn't always cause much, or any, pain, in which case a neurological disorder may be wrongly suspected. There may be no symptoms in the upper part of the body, so the possibility of a treatable spinal cord disease should be considered even in patients who present with symptoms confined to the legs.

Two inflammatory diseases that may cause neck pain are rheumatoid arthritis and ankylosing spondylitis. Radiographic evidence of forward displacement of the atlas on the axis is found in 30 per cent of patients with rheumatoid arthritis although this is not always associated with signs or symptoms. Ankylosing spondylitis may occasionally also produce subluxation of this kind.

Other, less usual, causes of neck pain include herpes zoster before the appearance of the rash, metastatic neoplasms, infections, metabolic bone diseases, and coronary artery ischaemia (cervical angina syndrome).

Physical examination

Pain in the neck may be precipitated by neck movements and there may be local tenderness and limitation of movement. We therefore first check the neck for range of movement in all planes: extension, rotation, and lateral tilting. Any restriction of movement is noted, and we try to estimate whether such restriction is due to muscular spasm or bony limitation. The first may be reduced by acupuncture whereas the second obviously will not.

We next make a detailed manual examination of the neck and shoulders for trigger points. These may be found anywhere, but the commonest sites are the trapezius muscle and the paraspinal muscles in the neck (splenius capitis, semispinalis capitis, longissimus capitis). Some degree of tenderness at the midpoint of the trapezius is to be expected, since this is a latent trigger point, but we need to decide whether the amount of tenderness present is more than would be expected for that patient. Women are usually more tender than men. If there is a difference between the two sides, this should be noted. If the tenderness is very marked the patient will flinch away from the examiner's fingers (jump sign).

Some patients have localized tenderness over the spines of the cervical or upper thoracic vertebrae, or over the interspinous ligament in these areas (type C pain).

Anteriorly, the sternocleidomastoid muscle is examined. A pincer action with finger and thumb is used for its lower part; nearer to its insertion at the base of the skull, direct pressure is used.

The radiation from these areas, and consequently the symptoms amenable to treatment by needling them, are variable. Radiation may be

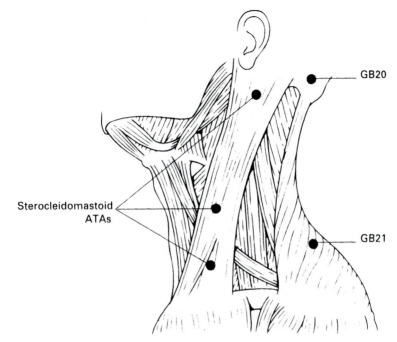

Muscles of the neck showing needling sites

downwards towards the shoulders and upper arms, or upwards, towards the face and head. Radiation to the head, particularly from the muscles of the neck, may extend over the scalp and forwards and downwards as far as the mouth.

Named acupuncture points

GB21 is a classic acupuncture point at the midpoint of the trapezius. It is one of the most frequently used sites in acupuncture. However, great precision is not required in needling here and one is guided by local tenderness as much as, or more than, by formal descriptions of where to needle. Often, anywhere in the trapezius muscle will have the same effect.

GB20 is a site at the base of the skull, lateral to the insertion of trapezius. It can be found by letting the fingers slip down over the back of the skull until they come off the nuchal ridge and sink into the muscles near their attachment.

'GB20.5' is not, of course, a classic acupuncture point, but it is a useful needling site. It is found at the junction between the neck and shoulders and is therefore situated in the levator scapulae muscle.

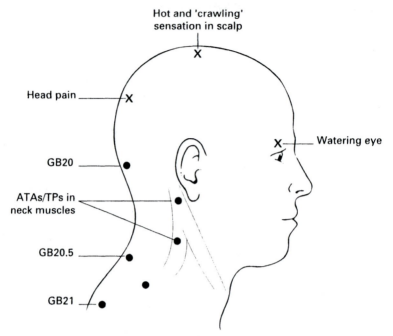

Needling points in neck and shoulders

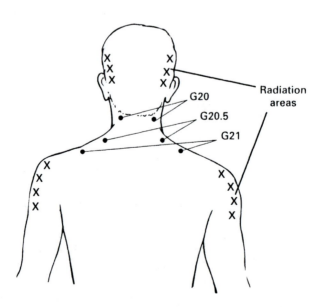

Needling sites in neck and shoulder, with characteristic radiation patterns

Positioning the patient for acupuncture

It's difficult to treat the shoulders with the patient lying down, partly because it makes some sites hard to reach and partly because, as noted in Chapter 7, it's desirable to have the muscles in slight stretch rather than totally relaxed. The patient should therefore ideally be seated, either on a stool or on a chair with a fairly low back, but if there is any fear that he will faint (particularly likely if he is a young fit man) he should sit on a couch with his back towards the acupuncturist; in this way, if a faint starts to occur it is easy to move him into a lying position.

However, as noted below, the base of the skull may be easier to needle if the patient lies prone and some people treat all the neck sites with the patient in this position.

Needling techniques

GB21 and GB20.5, possibly together with other tender areas in the trapezius muscles, can be needled easily, but it is important to keep the lung and pleura in mind. The needle should therefore be inserted in the anatomical horizontal plane. This means approximately parallel to the floor when the patient is sitting. The trapezius may be pinched up to make sure that the lung is avoided, and the needle is inserted either from a posterior or an anterior direction.

GB20 can be needled with the patient's head braced against the acupuncturist's chest to prevent movement. It is important to prevent the patient from looking downwards, since correct needling then becomes difficult or impossible. I generally insert the needle through the muscles and peck the underlying periosteum of the skull lightly. 'Lightly' is important, however, because although this point is very effective it is also one of the most likely sites to cause fainting.

An alternative, and preferable, position for treating GB20 is to have the patient lying prone, with no pillow or only a thin pillow, and the forehead resting on the hands, unless a couch with an aperture for the nose is available. The acupuncturist stands at the head of the couch. It is probably easier to needle the base of the skull with the patient in this position and it is also preferable if there is any possibility that the patient will faint.

The cervical muscles can be needled at sites of maximum tenderness. Relatively superficial needling is adequate, unless the aim is to needle the cervical periosteum (see below).

The sternocleidomastoid muscle can be needled wherever it is tender. In its lower part this should be done by holding the muscle between thumb and two fingers; in the upper part it is done directly into the muscle. A short needle may be preferable at these sites since there are numerous vulnerable vessels and nerves in the anterior triangle of the neck.

Indications

Headaches and migraines

'Classic migraine' ('migraine with aura') refers to headache associated with premonitory symptoms: these are typically visual but may be sensory or motor or may take the form of alterations in consciousness. There may be no headache but just the aura, which can make the diagnosis of migraine difficult ('migraine equivalent'). 'Common migraine' ('migraine without aura') is much the more frequent clinical form; here there is no warning but focal neurological disturbances may accompany the headache. So-called 'tension headache' is best regarded as common migraine, since there are no hard-and-fast criteria for distinguishing between them.

Acupuncture is frequently used for the treatment of headaches and appears to be successful in a good proportion of cases (about 75–80 per cent). The commonly used sites are the trapezius (GB21 and GB20.5) and also the base of the skull (GB20). The last-named is the most effective and would probably be enough by itself in many cases.

Acupuncture works best as a preventive, although it can sometimes abort a headache. It can also bring on a headache (aggravation). Note that acupuncture can relieve, temporarily, the headache of space-occupying lesions. This is an important reminder that acupuncture is a symptomatic treatment; the fact that a symptom is relieved by acupuncture should never be taken as an indication that there is no serious underlying pathology.

An alternative to needling the local areas in the shoulders and neck is to use generalized stimulation (LR3 – Chapter 15).

How to choose between local and generalized stimulation in headache

One should always look for trigger points in the head and neck, and these should generally be treated if they are present. However, LR3 can also work, and if it does it has certain advantages: it is quicker to perform and is something that patients can do for themselves if necessary (Chapter 18). Features that suggest trying LR3 first are a convincing history of headaches being precipitated by particular foods (chocolate, cheese) or alcohol, and the occurrence of a visual or other type of aura before the headaches. In other words, I think that LR3 is probably the first treatment to try for classic migraine and migraine triggered by food sensitivities, since these seem sometimes to diminish or disappear after acupuncture. It is also the treatment to try for migraine equivalent.

I would normally try both the head and neck and LR3 successively in migraine before giving up, since it isn't possible to be certain in advance about which is more likely to work. It might seem logical to try combined treatment in resistant cases, but in practice I haven't found that this helps if both approaches on their own have already failed.

Migraine in children

This should be treated at LR3; the results may be outstandingly good. I have seen two children aged under 10 who had migraine of great severity, so that they were unable to go to school most of the time; the headaches occurred two or three times weekly and were incapacitating. Acupuncture at LR3 in both cases, done very briefly (for a couple of seconds) gave prolonged relief, lasting for many months. These patients continued to attend about once a year for treatment until they were young adults.

I have a suspicion that acupuncture at LR3, if done during the aura phase of a migraine, can prolong the duration of the attack. This is based on only two cases, one of whom is myself.

> I get very occasional classic migraines; they occur about once or twice a year and are not of great severity. On one occasion I happened to have needles with me when the aura began. I tried needling LR3. The headache was of about the usual severity (i.e. not very severe and relieved by paracetamol), but it lasted for a full 24 hours, which is unusual for me; it usually finishes by the evening.

> I taught the father of a 16-year-old boy to treat his son, who suffered from migraine that was interfering with his school studies. This was pretty successful, but they reported that on one occasion when the acupuncture was done during the visual aura the subsequent headache lasted longer than usual.

Two classes of patients seldom respond to acupuncture. Women whose headaches occur close to or during menstruation often prove resistant (though headaches occurring at other times may improve). It may be worth trying the spleen points in such cases (see Chapter 13). Patients who have headaches every day also fail to respond as a rule. A common cause of chronic headaches in such cases is overuse of analgesics. Patients who take paracetamol daily for many months may suffer continuous headaches. In such cases the analgesics are producing the headaches and the only cure is to stop taking them. It is usually difficult to convince patients that the analgesics are responsible for their headaches, but if they can be persuaded to relinquish them they may experience dramatic relief. However, it's only fair to warn them that they will have six weeks of considerable suffering before the relief occurs. It is possible to withdraw the paracetamol gradually rather than suddenly but this is perhaps less effective.

Preparations containing ergotamine are sometimes used to relieve migraine but are even worse than paracetamol for precipitating headaches. Aspirin, however, does not appear to do this.

Cluster headaches

These almost never respond to acupuncture (although I have seen one patient who responded, but the history was unusual in this case).

Watering eye

Especially if unilateral and therefore unlikely to be allergic in nature, this may respond to needling GB20. Another idea is to needle periosteally around the orbit.

Psychological disorders

Patients who are anxious, depressed, or tense may have hard and tender shoulder muscles. Needling these muscles can relieve their symptoms, at least for a time. Although there are several classic acupuncture points that are recommended for anxiety, I have not found them to be any better than simple needling of the trapezius muscles (GB21). It is interesting that this point often figures in acupuncture cookbook 'recipes' for the treatment of a wide range of symptoms; presumably this reflects the fact that psychological tension is a contributing factor in many of these cases even when it is not the main cause.

Needling the trapezius seems to be particularly likely to set off an emotional abreaction in some patients, who may cry for some time after the acupuncture. It seems possible that in these cases longstanding psychological distress has led to chronic tension of the shoulder muscles, as if the patients were hunching themselves up as a protection against the unkind blows of fate. The muscular tension acts as a mask for inner unhappiness. Acupuncture seems to reverse this process in some way, so that as the tension in the muscles resolves the underlying psychological unhappiness reappears and causes the tears, although curiously the patients often do not seem to suffer much emotional distress. Similar effects can occur when other muscles are treated, though perhaps less frequently.

A possible explanation for these effects may be found in the ideas of the Austrian psychiatrist Wilhelm Reich (1897–1957), an associate of Freud. He postulated the existence of what he called 'muscular armour', by which he meant the set of chronic defensive attitudes a person adopts as a protection against personal injury (such as being hurt or rejected by others) and also against his or her own repressed emotions, especially rage and anxiety. For example, anxiety is reflected in the hunching of the shoulders, rage in a tight chin, disgust in a certain habitual expression of the mouth, and so on. It is a mistake, he believed, to regard the muscular rigidity as a mere accompaniment or an effect of the corresponding character attitude; it is its 'somatic side and the basis for its continuing existence'.

In his later years in the USA Reich developed other ideas, notably about orgone (an energy that is supposed to permeate the cosmos and to possess healing powers, rather reminiscent of qi), and eventually he became progressively eccentric and even paranoid; however, his 'muscular armour' theory seems to me to be genuinely illuminating.

Other disorders associated with radiation effects

As noted above, there may be triggers in the neck muscles which are relevant to neck pain and other symptoms. It is difficult to specify these symptoms in detail because they are so variable. One pattern seen quite often in elderly patients is creeping or crawling sensations on top of the head. These can be relieved by needling tender areas in the posterior neck muscles. Other radiation effects may also occur.

A man in his early 40s came with a complaint of pain in the root of his tongue, which troubled him mostly at night. He had been investigated by a dentist and an ear, nose, and throat surgeon but no cause had been found. He had a trigger zone near the insertion of the sternocleidomastoid on the affected side; needling this on a few occasions relieved his pain completely.

Needling the cervical articular column

In many cases it is enough to needle the posterior or lateral neck muscles (splenius capitis, scalene muscles) for localized pain and also to obtain radiation effects. However, by needling a little deeper it is possible to reach the periosteum of the cervical articular column. This is a major ATA that is capable of influencing a wide range of symptoms in the upper half of the body as well as local neck problems (Russ *et al.*, 1999).

Although this treatment is safe if done carefully, it requires a good knowledge of anatomy and should not be attempted in people with thick necks. In such cases, or if the acupuncturist is not confident about performing the treatment safely, ordinary needling of the musculature should be used instead. Note that the articular column is not the same as the transverse processes of the vertebrae; these are situated anterior to the column. It is essential to study the anatomy carefully before attempting this treatment and the acupuncturist should look at an articulated skeleton as well as at diagrams in books; as with most acupuncture treatments, practical instruction is essential before one undertakes it.

The treatment may be done with the patient sitting but it is easier to place them prone, with the head resting on the hands or on a pillow, as for needling G20. The spine is then palpated at the C3 or C4 level. The tissues

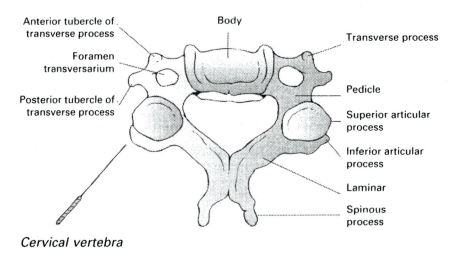

Cervical vertebra

are compressed with the free hand and a fine needle is then inserted at about 45 degrees to the midline plane. The periosteum will be reached within a short distance (about 5 mm in a suitably thin patient) and it is pecked gently two or three times. If the periosteum has not been reached after the needle has penetrated to this depth, it indicates that the angle was incorrect and the needle has missed the articular column; no attempt to needle more deeply should be made. In obese patients or in men who are very heavily muscled, only the overlying tissues should be needled.

Mann, who first described this technique (Mann, 2000), uses it in a wide range of disorders and symptom complexes affecting the upper half of the body, and my experience of its efficacy agrees with his. I regard it as the best treatment to try for carpal tunnel syndrome, which often responds provided it is not too severe. It can also be used for autonomic disturbances of the hands, including Raynaud's disease.

A woman in her 70s, a keen amateur bridge player, was unable to hold the cards because of pain in her hands, which she described as resembling hot swollen cushions. They were indeed red and swollen. She had consulted a neurologist and a rheumatologist without receiving any help. The main finding on examination, apart from the redness of her hands, was limitation of movement in her neck, presumably due to spondylosis. I therefore needled the cervical articular column bilaterally and also needled the interosseus muscles in her hands (this is described in Chapter 11). Within two or three treatments the pain in her hands had gone and their appearance had returned to normal. Although she continued to need treatment for her neck and lumbar spine in subsequent years (to which she always responded very well), she had no recurrence of the hand problem over a number of years.

Needling the cervical articular column can relieve the symptoms of mild vertigo or unsteadiness quite frequently seen in elderly patients. Such patients are often told they have vertebrobasilar artery insufficiency. This seems an unlikely explanation for their symptoms, since obstruction of the vertebral artery, which supplies the brain stem, would be more likely to cause unconsciousness than giddiness. There are several possible causes for this giddiness, but in many instances the probable explanation is disease of the facet joints in the neck. The innervation of these joints is closely connected with the vestibular apparatus in the brain stem and forms part of the proprioceptive balance mechanism. When this is disturbed, as it is by disease of the facet joints, this can give rise to abnormal information about body position when the patient turns his or her head. Needling the periosteum in this area, or failing that, needling the neck muscles, can give relief lasting for about 12 weeks each time it is done. However, it is unlikely to help in Ménière's disease or other kinds of vertigo, so it is important to take a detailed history; further investigations may be needed in some cases.

Tinnitus is normally unresponsive to acupuncture. However, I have seen occasional patients in whom the tinnitus came on after road traffic injuries in which the neck was violently stretched. In these cases there were trigger points in the neck muscles, and needling these eliminated the tinnitus. I have also seen one patient in whom needling the neck gave a temporary improvement in hearing. He was partially deaf as a result of blast exposure during the war. The acupuncture was being performed for neck symptoms, not deafness, but his wife noticed an improvement in his hearing, lasting for about four days after each treatment.

The face

Deep infratemporal fossa (DIF)

This is an important ATA for the treatment of trigeminal neuralgia. Although the site could be needled with the patient sitting, I generally work with the patient lying on their side, with the side to be needled uppermost. The side of the face is palpated and the inferior border of the zygomatic arch is identified. This border is traced backwards until the anterior border of the ramus of the mandible is encountered; it is felt rather indistinctly owing to the overlying masseter muscle. The angle between these two bones forms the landmark for needling. A fine 30-mm needle is inserted and passed slightly upwards and slightly backwards, to a depth of about 20 mm. In some cases the maxilla will be touched by the needle tip; this does no harm but the treatment is not intended to be periosteal. The needle is stimulated manually as usual for about 20 seconds and then withdrawn. Patients hardly ever find this a painful procedure. I generally treat both sides because this seems to give better results than treating only one side.

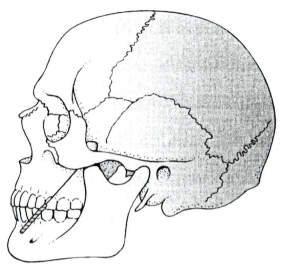

Needling the deep infratemporal fossa

Success rates are quite good: about 65 per cent response rates, with the treatment being repeated whenever necessary to maintain the remission. Relief is not always complete but is often worthwhile, with a reduction in the need for medication. Very severe pain is not usually helped and, if the face is anaesthetic as a result of previous nerve block, needling will not work. (It is possible to treat the opposite side in such cases but this seldom helps.)

Some patients are left with residual pain, perhaps in a line along the angle of the jaw; in these, I sometimes insert some short needles subcutaneously over the area of pain.

Atypical facial pain is more difficult to help than true trigeminal neuralgia and seldom responds to the same treatment. Local needling over the painful area may be tried in such cases.

Other ATAs in the face

The periosteum over the frontal bone and over the maxillae on each side constitutes another ATA, which is relevant to recurrent sneezing. The classic acupuncture points in this area are BL2 and ST2. Patients who wake up in the morning and sneeze repeatedly are often helped by needling at these sites. Almost all patients in whom this is done will report an immediate clearing of the nasal passages. Such needling can also help in chronic sinusitis, though the results are less impressive. It is important to realize that many patients who have been diagnosed as suffering from chronic sinusitis don't actually have sinus inflammation; they are suffering from referred pain from their neck region, which radiates forward to the front of the head and mimics sinusitis.

The classic acupuncture point LI4, in the web between the first and second metacarpal bones, is supposed to be related to sinus symptoms. However, I have seldom been convinced that it adds greatly to the success rate, and it may also be more likely to be responsible for adverse effects than most other sites (see Chapter 15).

Infra-orbital nerve (almost B2): this emerges from the infraorbital foramen and divides into branches, which run over the anterior surface of the maxilla. Needling these branches in a little arc below the foramen will nearly always turn off the twitching that characterizes the disorder known as clonic facial spasm (facial myoclonus). This is a motor disorder of unknown cause; it is not the same as blepharospasm. It is unilateral and is the only dystonia I know of that responds to acupuncture. Neurologists seem to be uncertain whether it is mainly psychological or mainly organic; in the patients I have seen it is made worse by psychological tension but this probably isn't the primary cause. One patient had himself discovered that pressing over the nerve with a pencil would stop the spasms. Acupuncture is certainly helpful in the short term but it may be difficult to get sustained relief; in one case the patient was able to achieve this by using a TENS machine over the site every day.

References

Mann F. (2000) Reinventing acupuncture: a new concept of ancient medicine. Butterworth-Heinemann, Oxford.

Ross J. *et al.* (1999) Western minimal acupuncture for neck pain: a cohort study. *Acupuncture in Medicine*, 17: 5–8.

Chapter 10

The shoulder

Pain in or around the shoulder is often a difficult diagnostic problem, since it may arise from the shoulder structures themselves or be referred to the shoulder from elsewhere. The acupuncture treatment will naturally vary according to the source of the pain.

Pain arising outside the shoulder

As noted in the previous chapter, neck disorders can cause pain that radiates to the shoulder or down the arm. Pain of this kind can also be caused by the thoracic outlet syndrome and by various neurological disorders.

Thoracic outlet syndrome

There are at least three varieties of the thoracic outlet syndrome, in two of which the mechanism is clear-cut. Compression of the lower trunk of the plexus is due to an anomalous band of tissue connecting an elongated transverse process of C7 to the first rib. It produces neurological changes in the hand and the diagnosis is confirmed by electromyography and by nerve conduction studies. The second type is due to compression of the subclavian artery by a cervical rib; there are no neurological signs but thrombosis may occur in the artery. Doppler techniques confirm the diagnosis. Acupuncture is unsuitable for treating either of these forms, which require surgery if they are causing symptoms.

The third group (the 'disputed thoracic outlet syndrome') includes a large number of patients with chronic arm and shoulder pain of unknown cause. There are no definite abnormalities on physical examination and laboratory investigations are unhelpful. Treatment in this group is correspondingly difficult, and these are patients in whom acupuncture may be worth trying. (A case of thoracic outlet syndrome successfully treated with acupuncture has recently been reported by Tariq *et al.*, 2000).

Disorders affecting the brachial plexus and peripheral nerves

Injury to these structures, for example due to infiltration of the nerves by neoplasm, may cause shoulder pain radiating down the arm, together with numbness of the fourth and fifth fingers and weakness of intrinsic muscles innervated by the ulnar and median nerves. Post-radiation fibrosis may also do this, and so may a Pancoast tumour of the lung (generally in association with Horner's syndrome). Suprascapular neuropathy gives rise to pain, weakness, and wasting of the supraspinatus and infraspinatus muscles.

A disorder often confused with radiculopathy is acute brachial neuritis, in which there is acute onset of shoulder pain, followed after some days or weeks by weakness of the proximal arm and shoulder girdle. The cause is unknown although previous infection or immunization has been blamed. Most patients recover completely in two to three years.

Occasionally, carpal tunnel syndrome may give pain and paraesthesiae extending proximally up to the shoulder.

Mechanical shoulder pain

Few of the preceding causes of pain are likely to be suitable for acupuncture. It may, however, be tried for mechanical shoulder pain.

Unfortunately, mechanical shoulder pain may be difficult to distinguish from other types. If symptoms and signs of radiculopathy are not found the diagnosis of mechanical shoulder pain becomes more probable, although the possibility of referral (from subdiaphragmatic irritation, a Pancoast tumour, or angina) must be remembered. Clinical features that suggest mechanical pain include pain that is worse at night, local shoulder tenderness, and pain made worse by particular arm movements (abduction, internal rotation, or extension). Although the pain may radiate to the arm or hand there are no sensory, motor, or reflex changes.

Mechanical shoulder pain is often labelled as 'frozen shoulder': an unsatisfactory term, which really serves to conceal our substantial ignorance about what is really going on. (As T.D. Bunker (1985) remarked, no one would accept 'frozen knee' as a valid diagnosis, so why do we accept 'frozen shoulder'?) 'Frozen shoulder' should in any case not be accepted as a diagnosis without further investigations. Dr Virginia Camp, a rheumatologist who uses acupuncture, found in the course of five years 12 patients with a diagnosis of frozen shoulder who had serious underlying disease: eight had cancers of various kinds and had had leukaemia (Camp, 1986).

It is customary to distinguish two varieties of shoulder disease: intrinsic and extrinsic. Intrinsic disease is thought to be due to capsulitis (adhesive capsulitis). This is generally unilateral, though sometimes the opposite shoulder is affected later. It is not part of a generalized arthritis and the cause is unknown. It generally resolves over one to two years, although there may be some residual restriction of movement which is permanent. Sometimes there is a prodromal period of mild aching; this is followed by increasing pain and stiffness, until almost no movement at all is possible in the shoulder joint, although scapular mobility allows for a certain amount of arm movement. The pain is often worse at night and may be very severe. The pain then diminishes slowly, and finally the range of movement begins to increase. Clinical examination during the first two phases shows movements in all planes, both active and passive, to be restricted or completely inhibited.

Extrinsic shoulder disease is due to damage to the structures round the joint, especially the rotator cuff, made up of the supraspinatus, infraspinatus, teres minor, and subscapularis muscles, which have a conjoint tendinous insertion into the humerus and act both as lateral rotators and abductors of the humerus. Lesions in these structures are often not induced by trauma but are due to degenerative avascular necrosis. This may occur spontaneously or following some unusual activity. It can occur at any age but is commonest in the 40s and 50s. Unlike the total restriction of movement found in capsulitis, only certain movements are painful and resisted movement may hurt whereas passive movements are pain-free. The 'painful arc' syndrome is characterized by impingement of the acromion on the supraspinatus tendon when the arm is abducted beyond a certain point. Partial or complete tears of the rotator cuff tendons also occur, often following quite minor stress on a tendon that is already weakened by degenerative changes. Minor tears heal spontaneously but more severe tears may require surgery.

Acupuncture treatment of the shoulder

The main periosteal needling sites in the shoulder are the coracoid process and the lesser tuberosity of the humerus, both of which are at least latent trigger points. These are most conveniently needled with the patient sitting.

There are also numerous soft-tissue sites in the shoulder muscles. These may lie in the anterior or posterior axillary folds (pectoralis major and minor; subscapularis, teres major, teres minor, infraspinatus). To needle these, the fold is gripped between finger and thumb (pincer action) and the muscles are palpated for trigger points, into which the needle is then inserted.

Yet another useful needling site is the area above the tendon of supraspinatus as it passes over the top of the humerus beneath the acromion. The needle is inserted posterolaterally, between the acromion and the top of the humerus at an angle of about 45 degrees to the sagittal plane; this is much the same approach as that commonly used to inject the shoulder. It is particularly indicated for patients who show the painful arc phenomenon.

Mann identifies two further sites (Mann, 2000), which he calls Hansen 1 and Hansen 2. (The name refers to a Dr Hansen, from whom he learned these sites.) Hansen 1 is 2 or 3 cm below the medial third of the scapula, in the fibres of trapezius; it approximately corresponds to SI11 but is medial to it. Hansen 2 is the infraglenoid tubercle, to which the long head of the triceps is attached. This point is notably tender in almost everyone (latent trigger point). It is most conveniently needled with the patient lying down, slightly rotated towards the opposite side, and with the fingers of the affected arm touching the opposite shoulder. The point cannot be clearly identified unless the patient is slim; in fatter patients only superficial acupuncture should be attempted.

On the whole, one's enthusiasm for treating shoulder pain with acupuncture needs to be tempered with caution. Acupuncture may on occasion help with both intrinsic and extrinsic shoulder pain but the success rate is not high; perhaps one-third of those with intrinisic pain will respond. As was pointed out some time ago by H. Berry and others (Berry *et al.*, 1980), similar proportions of patients respond to other available forms of treatment and also to no treatment at all! Even when acupuncture is successful, it generally relieves pain for a time without altering the natural course of the disease, which as noted above is towards recovery within one to two years. However, occasional patients do respond dramatically so acupuncture is always worth trying.

Patients should be advised about preventive measures. Posture may contribute to rotator cuff tendinitis; avoid working above shoulder level, because the supraspinatus tendon is forced under the coraco-acromial arch during elevation of the arm. Reduced blood flow to the tendons due to static muscle contraction may contribute to tendon degeneration. Repetitive movement of the shoulder may cause rotator cuff tendinitis.

Osteoarthritic pain in the shoulder region, arising either from the glenohumeral or acromioclavicular joints, usually does poorly with acupuncture.

Chest pain referred from chest wall muscles

Trigger points in the pectoralis major muscle are relevant to cardiac pain due to angina pectoris. There are tender areas in these muscles in people without angina, but in patients with angina pressure at these sites can produce long-lasting, severe pain. This may be a summation effect, whereby pain information arising from two different structures (pectoralis major and heart muscle) is added together centrally to give rise the conscious experience of pain. It is sometimes possible to relieve angina by needling these trigger points, although the possibility of precipitating a severe anginal attack has to be kept in mind. There is also a question about the desirability of relieving angina in this way, since the cardiac flow rate is presumably not improved. Most doctors, at least in Britain, regard angina as a warning sign telling the patient to stop doing whatever has brought on the pain, and if this is correct (some cardiologists dispute it), relieving angina by acupuncture would be ill-advised except in those few patients who fail to respond to medical or surgical treatment, for whom it may be useful.

The similarity between chest pain due to trigger points in the muscles and chest pain due to angina can pose a difficult problem in diagnosis. Both types of pain may be brought on by exertion, but skeletal pain may be aggravated by stretching and twisting movements. A therapeutic trial of medication doesn't distinguish between the two types of pain reliably because there is a considerable placebo response. An electrocardiogram may not give the answer either. In some cases it may be necessary to resort to sophisticated cardiological investigations to make the diagnosis.

> A woman had been admitted to hospital on several occasions with suspected cardiac pain but nothing was found to confirm the diagnosis. She had numerous trigger points in her pectoralis major and subscapularis muscles and needling these prevented further episodes of pain.

References

Berry H. *et al.* (1980) Clinical study comparing acupuncture, physiotherapy, injections and oral anti-inflammatory drugs in shoulder cuff lesions. *Current Medical Research Opinion*, 7; 121–6.

Bunker T.D. (1985) Time for a new name for 'frozen shoulder'. *British Medical Journal*, 291; 1233.

Camp V. (1986) Acupuncture for shoulder pain. *Acupuncture in Medicine*, 3; 28–32.

Mann F. (2000) *Reinventing Acupuncture: a new concept of ancient medicine* (second edition). Butterworth-Heinemann, London.

Tariq M. *et al.* (2000) Role of acupuncture in thoracic outlet syndrome. *Acupuncture in Medicine*, 18; 122–3.

Chapter 11

The upper limb

The elbow

Like the shoulder, the elbow can be difficult to help with acupuncture. Remember the possibility that elbow pain is being referred from the neck; this is probably quite common. The neck should therefore always be examined in patients with elbow pain, and even if nothing definite is found, the cervical articular column (Chapter 9) can be treated as an ATA that may radiate to the elbow.

Many patients come with a diagnosis of 'tennis elbow' or 'golfer's elbow'. In these disorders, pain is felt at the lateral or medial elbow areas respectively, and there is usually exquisite tenderness over the common tendon origin of the affected muscles at the lateral or medial epicondyle of the humerus. It isn't only tennis players or golfers who may be affected; any repetitive movement, such as removing bottle tops, may give rise to pain of this kind. Pain at the lateral epicondyle is commoner and more troublesome, as a rule, than pain at the medial epicondyle.

So-called tennis elbow and golfer's elbow are usually treated conventionally by injection of corticosteroids plus a local anaesthetic into the common tendon origin. Although standard textbooks recommend this treatment, P.E. Baldry has pointed out that there is rather little information available about the proportion of patients that can be expected to respond, and he is not convinced that this treatment is particularly effective (Baldry, 1998). There is also uncertainty about whether the injection should be given into the periosteum. At least one study has found that acupuncture was twice as effective as corticosteroid injection for this purpose. The advantage of acupuncture is that it can be repeated as many times as necessary. There is thus a good case to be made for trying plain needling of the common tendon origin a few times before resorting to local hydrocortisone injection. However, it's often the lot of the acupuncturist to see only those patients in whom previous hydrocortisone injection has failed, and this has been my own experience. In these cases there is nothing to be gained by needling the same site and one needs to try something different.

The alternative approach consists in looking for trigger points in the muscles around the elbow. Any muscles may be affected; they include the medial border of the triceps, the supinator, the brachioradialis, and extensor carpi radialis longus. These, however, are just general guidelines, not inflexible rules, and the treatment depends on making a careful examination of all the muscles in the region and needling those that are found to be tender.

Intrinsic elbow disease, due, for example, to 'burnt-out' rheumatoid arthritis, may respond to the standard acupuncture joint treatment of periosteal needling, which is conveniently done by needling the lower part of the shaft of the humerus on the lateral side (well below the radial nerve) and the border of the ulna below the olecranon.

A woman had had rheumatoid arthritis for many years. It was now relatively inactive but she still had considerable pain in her elbows. They were semi-ankylosed, so that she had only about 15 degrees of movement. Needling the shaft of the humerus and the border of the ulna gave her relief of pain lasting for 12 weeks on each occasion, though the range of movement was not of course increased. The treatment continued to be effective over a period of more than eight years.

Muscles of the forearm

The muscles in this region are an important site of trigger points, which may radiate symptoms either proximally, to the elbow, or distally, or the wrist and hand. There are numerous muscles in the region that may be relevant.

Anteriorly there are superficial and deep groups. The superficial group is made up of pronator teres, flexor carpi radialis, flexor carpi ulnaris, flexor digitorum sublimis, and palmaris longus (if present); the deep group contains flexor digitorum profundus, flexor pollicis longus, and pronator quadratus.

Posteriorly there are again superficial and deep groups. The superficial group has seven muscles (brachioradialis, extensor digitorum, extensor carpi radialis longus, extensor carpi radialis brevis, extensor digiti minimi, extensor carpi ulnaris, and anconeus); the deep group has five (supinator, extensor pollicis brevis, abductor pollicis longus, extensor pollicis longus, and extensor indicis).

Classic acupuncture points in the area are LU5, PC3, HT3; SI8, LI8–LI12. However, I shall disregard these and instead simply refer to the anterior forearm ATA and the posterior forearm ATA. There are often trigger areas in these muscles but the ATAs may, as usual, be needled even when there is no definite tenderness.

Anterior forearm ATA

Trigger points in this region may cause weakness of the hands.

> A middle-aged man who worked in an engineering department, where he had to carry heavy machinery in his hands, found he was dropping things. Multiple sclerosis had been suspected but was excluded. Needling the anterior forearm muscles restored his strength. He returned for further treatment after a year but was not seen again after that. What seems to have happened in this case is that declining strength with advancing age had made him more liable to develop trigger points in his flexor muscles; these were eliminated by acupuncture.

Triggers in the anterior forearm ATA may cause elbow pain and needling here helps in about one-third of cases.

Some patients with writer's cramp have trigger points in the flexor muscles of the forearm, and in these cases acupuncture may help. As a rule, however, writer's cramp is a form of motor dystonia and does not respond to acupuncture.

Pain in the base of the thumb is sometimes helped by needling in this area.

Posterior forearm ATA

There is nearly always a latent trigger in the portion of extensor digitorum that operates the middle finger. 'Plucking' this strand of muscle, as if it were a guitar string, often causes a twitch. Activation of this trigger may give rise to pain in the dorsum of the wrist, which may be surprisingly localized, perhaps to an area only a few millimetres across. Overuse of the fingers, as in typing, can be the cause. Acupuncture may relieve the pain very effectively, but it needs to be done accurately. The strand of affected muscles is identified by palpation, and then the needle is passed in obliquely, so as to transfix as much of the muscle as possible. If the affected region is penetrated accurately the patient is likely to experience the needle as if it were quite thick, and sensations may travel down the arm to the wrist. This is then followed by improvement and sometimes permanent remission of symptoms.

On the lateral side there are ATAs in the muscles, brachioradialis and the extensor group, including the long muscles of the thumb. Logically, one would expect treating these to be relevant to pain in the thumb, and to a certain extent it is; but I have generally found thumb pain to be difficult to treat. It is unclear why this should be so, considering that the results of treating the big toe are so good. Other needling sites for the thumb are LI4, between the first and second metatarsal bones, the lower end of the radius and the shaft of the first metacarpal bone.

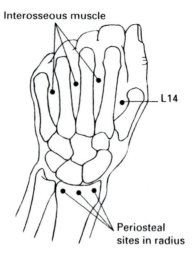

Acupuncture sites on hand and wrist

Wrist and hand

Intrinsic wrist pain, for example due to osteoarthritis, may be helped in many cases by needling the lower end of the radius periosteally at two or three sites.

Nausea and vomiting: PC6

The classic acupuncture point known as PC6 is found at the front of the wrist. This is an anti-nausea treatment site and is probably the best-researched classic acupuncture point in the body. A number of controlled trials have been carried out since the mid-1980s, almost all of which have confirmed the efficacy of this site for the control of nausea and vomiting due to drugs or anaesthetics; the present position has been well reviewed by C.M. McMillan (1998). I have not found it to be useful for vomiting associated with migraine but it was remarkably successful in a particularly severe case of vomiting from unknown cause.

PC6 is situated 2 *cun* above the distal skin crease at the wrist, between the tendons of flexor carpi radialis and palmaris longus (this assumes that palmaris longus is present, which is not always the case). A *cun* may be taken to be the width of the thumb across the interphalangeal joint. It's quite easy to hit the median nerve while needling this site unless the depth of penetration is closely controlled; it produces a sharp electric-shock sensation that radiates into the hand, but the effect is seldom long-lasting. As an alternative to needling, simple pressure may be used. 'Sea Bands' are available for purchase and are used for travel sickness, although the same effect may be achieved by fixing a bead in place with a piece of adhesive strapping.

A woman suffered from amoebic dysentery while on holiday in India and began to vomit repeatedly. She was treated for the dysentery but the vomiting didn't abate. She returned to Britain and was extensively investigated. A peptic ulcer was found and treated but the vomiting continued; by this time she was becoming seriously ill and had lost a lot of weight. A brain tumour was sought but not found. She then turned up at our outpatient department. I tried LR3, but 10 days later she was no better. I therefore admitted her to hospital; the anti-emetic effect of PC6 had recently been reported at this time, so we placed stud needles in this site bilaterally and gave her continuous electrical stimulation via a TENS machine. Over the next three or four days her vomiting cleared up and she was discharged. She returned with a relapse after a month; we repeated the treatment and she again responded, with no further recurrence.

A number of general practitioners currently use PC6 for treating nausea of pregnancy and report good results; it appears to be safe for this purpose. However, a recent randomized controlled trial found acupuncture to be equivalent to a sham procedure using a cocktail stick (Knight, 2001). The acupuncture in question was the traditional form, using pulse and tongue diagnosis. PC6 was needled, together with a number of other points chosen in accordance with the traditional theory. Sham treatment consisted in tapping a blunt cocktail stick over a bony prominence in the region of each acupuncture point. Both treatments gave good symptomatic relief and the researchers conclude that the effect was probably due to placebo response.

Pain in the hands, especially osteoarthritic hand pain

The interosseus muscles constitute a major ATA for the treatment of hand pain, especially that due to osteoarthritis of the type found in postmenopausal women and associated with the development of Heberden's nodes. This is probably one of the most effective acupuncture treatments. The muscles may be treated by directing the needle obliquely between the metacarpal bones in each interspace. Patients generally experience pain relief lasting 8–12 weeks after each treatment.

Travell and Simons, who describe a similar treatment consisting in the injection of local anaesthetic into these areas, claim that it may cause Heberden's nodes to disappear (Travell & Simons, 1983). This seemed unlikely to me when I first read about it, but over the years I have had a number of patients report that their nodes have, in fact, become smaller.

The classic acupuncture site LI4

The space between the thumb and first finger is a special site, known in the classic system as LI4. It is supposed to be useful for sinusitis and also for dental pain. I have not generally found it to be useful for sinusitis and I have only very limited experience of using it for dental pain. I tend to regard it as a site of generalized stimulation, analogous to LR3, but probably less effective. Nowadays I use it infrequently, in spite of its prominence in the recipes of traditional acupuncture. In part this is because I think it is more likely to cause adverse effects than some other sites (see Chapter 4).

Pain in interphalangeal joints

Pain in individual fingers may be treated in the usual way, by periosteal needling. The shafts of the phalanges should be needled above and below the affected joints; this is done obliquely, so as to avoid penetrating the extensor tendons.

> A man suffering from Reiter's syndrome had swelling and pain of his right middle first metacarpal joint. This was a particular problem for him because he was a keen amateur guitarist. Acupuncture to the interosseus muscles and to the shaft of his middle finger relieved the pain and reduced his swelling by about a half; he was then able to play the guitar. Repeat treatments were needed at intervals of about 9–12 months.

Trigger finger: this is due to a constriction of one of the sheaths of the digital flexor tendons in the palm; when the finger is flexed it becomes locked and has to be straightened with the other hand. There is usually a very tender spot in the palm just proximal to the head of the metacarpal bone, which can be needled with good effect.

Overuse syndrome: repetitive strain injury (RSI)

This diagnosis became fashionable in the late 1980s and early 1990s and we started seeing a lot of patients suffering from such symptoms at this time in our clinics, especially affecting musicians and typists. I felt fairly confident that we should be able to help them by means of acupuncture, since I assumed that the cause was active trigger points in the relevant muscles. Alas, not so; there were some successes, but most of the patients did badly. I was puzzled and disappointed, but later some information appeared which may shed light on my failure. There is now some evidence that severe RSI is a form of dystonia, analogous to writer's cramp (Byl *et al.*, 1997; Bara-Jimenez *et al.*, 1998; Candia *et al.*, 1999;

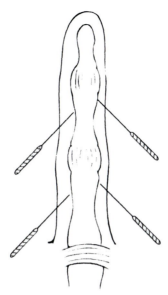

Needling sites on sides and shaft of finger

Holmes, 1999). We already know that the sensory map in the cortex is not fixed but plastic – capable of rapid change in response to painful stimuli (see Chapter 3). Now the suggestion is that this may also happen in RSI. Repetitive movements of the hand may cause 'smearing' of the maps in both the sensory and motor cortices. In normal people, the cortical sensory zones for the thumb and the little finger are about 12 mm apart, but in patients with severe RSI they may overlap almost completely. Similar effects have been found in the thalamus of affected musicians.

The suggested treatment in these cases is exercises to retrain the sensory and motor systems. Patients have been asked to identify letters or numbers blindfold, and have been given exercises for the affected fingers with the unaffected fingers splinted. These measures have produced improvements.

This work is still at an early stage. We don't know if the improvements that have been found are a placebo effect, and it's unknown why only certain people become affected; not all musicians suffer symptoms of this kind. Is this because of a genetic predisposition, or is it caused by differences in the way they hold their instruments? We also don't know exactly how these central changes occur. One idea is that repetitive use of muscles may activate sensory connections that are usually suppressed.

Although the research to date has focused on musicians and others suffering from severe RSI, there is speculation that the effect may exist in many types of chronic pain in which there is no obvious local pathology. I once spent a day working with two physiotherapists who had done my acupuncture course and who were involved in the treatment of ballet dancers. They told me that the dancers tended to fall into two groups: one group had few or no symptoms, while the other had repeated musculoskeletal problems. Conceivably this pattern is similar to what is found among musicians.

If these findings are confirmed, they would help to explain why my results using acupuncture to treat musicians with RSI were mostly unsatisfactory. Acupuncture generally does not work for dystonias. As usual, however, one needs to be cautious about accepting the diagnostic labels that patients arrive with. I have seen some people who were diagnosed as having writer's cramp, but the symptoms were not typical and, on examining them, I found definite triggers in their arms and shoulders which are absent in true writer's cramp. Needling these sites relieved their symptoms. The moral of this is that what matters is what you find on examination, not the formal diagnosis the patient has been given previously, which may be wrong.

References

Baldry P.E. (1998) *Acupuncture, Trigger Points and Musculoskeletal Pain*. Churchill Livingstone, Edinburgh.

Bara-Jimenez W. *et al.* (1998) Abnormal somatosensory homunculus in dystonia of the hand. *Annals of Neurology* 44; 828.

Byl N. *et al.* (1997) A primate model for studying focal dystonia and repetitive strain injury, *Physical Therapy*, 77; 269.

Candia V. *et al.* (1999) Constraint-induced movement therapy for focal hand dystonia in musicians. *Lancet*, 353; 42.

Holmes B. (1999) The strain is in the brain. *New Scientist*, 10 April.

Knight B. *et al.* (2001) Effect of acupuncture on nausea of pregnancy: a randomized, controlled trial. *Obstetrics and Gynaecology*, 97; 184–8.

McMillan C.M. (1998) Acupuncture for nausea and vomiting. In: *Medical Acupuncture: a Western scientific approach* (eds Filshie J. & White A.). Churchill Livingstone, Edinburgh.

Travell J.G. & Simons D.G. (1983) *Myofascial Pain and Dysfunction. The trigger point manual*, Vol. 1. Williams & Wilkins, Baltimore.

Chapter 12

The thoracic and lumbar spine

Thoracic spine

Needling over the thoracic spine must be carried out carefully owing to the presence of the spinal cord at this level. Superficial needling over the tips of the spinous processes and interspinous ligament for localized pain is safe, though it is best done with short needles to make sure that there is no danger of reaching the cord.

Pain in the chest wall often occurs for unknown reasons. This can be treated by local needling over the site of pain; of course, the needles should be inserted at a shallow angle to avoid causing a pneumothorax. There is no need to try to needle the intercostal muscles, and indeed this would be dangerous.

Persistent pain in a rib, due to trauma or fracture, responds well to periosteal pecking at the site of tenderness. To do this, fix the rib between two of your fingers to make sure that you do not inadvertently penetrate the pleura. This treatment should not be attempted in an obese patient.

There is a distant point that sometimes seems to help with thoracic pain; this is SI3 at the ulnar side of the hand. It is one of the few remote sites for pain that I have found to be useful. The needle is passed transversely across the palm, in front of the fifth metacarpal. This is a painful treatment and it is likely that in many cases the same effect would be produced, with less pain, by needling the space between the fourth and fifth metacarpals from the dorsal surface (this is approximately TE3).

The sternum

There is a classic acupuncture point (CV17) which is situated over the lower part of the body of the sternum, at the level of the fifth costal cartilages. It is often recommended for respiratory problems but in my experience is generally ineffective for these; however, it can be used for patients who have non-cardiac pain in the centre of the chest. Other regions of the sternum are often treated at the same time (CV18–CV20).

Of course, when treating these areas it is essential to remember the potentially lethal sternal defect that may lead to cardiac tamponade (see Chapter 4); the needle must therefore be inserted tangentially to the sternum so that there is no risk of penetrating it.

Tietze's syndrome, in which there is pain and swelling of one or more costal cartilages, can be treated by pecking the affected costal cartilages; this is similar to the conventional treatment, which consists in local infiltration with a corticosteroid, but it has the advantage that it can be repeated as many times as necessary.

Widespread spinal pain

Patients who have pain throughout much of the spine, due, for example, to ankylosing spondylitis or osteoporosis, often respond to acupuncture. This consists simply in placing a number of needles (perhaps a dozen or more) in the paraspinal muscles throughout the painful area, which may include the whole thoracic and lumbar spine. There is no need to search for triggers in the muscles; simply put the needles in at roughly 2 cm intervals. I usually do this in a zigzag pattern, starting at the top, using medium-length (30 mm) needles. All the needles are put in; each is given a brief manual stimulation and then they are all withdrawn. The total treatment takes about 3 minutes, and pain relief on each occasion usually lasts for about 12 weeks.

Low back pain and sciatica

Pain in the lumbar spine and referred pain to the legs are symptoms that often fall to acupuncturists to treat, which is not surprising in view of how widespread they are. The incidence seems to be increasing; in Britain during the ten years up to 1993, outpatient attendances for this reason rose fivefold and the number of days for which social security was paid more than doubled. However, this may be due to a greater willingness on the part of patients to report symptoms rather than to a true increase in the number of patients suffering in this way, since the incidence of disabling back pain has not changed; the increase has been in back disorders that don't significantly impair spinal flexion. This suggests that there is a cultural element in people's attitudes to back pain.

Acute or chronic?

Acute back pain is defined as pain of less than 3 months' duration, although in practice most patients in the 'acute' category recover considerably sooner than 3 months. Full recovery can be expected in 85 per cent of patients whose back pain is not accompanied by leg pain.

Acupuncture can certainly be used in the acute phase, but there is no firm evidence to show that it shortens the duration of pain and disability. (The same is true of other forms of treatment.) Acupuncture is more often used for chronic pain, here defined as pain lasting more than 12 weeks.

Chronic back pain is of great economic importance: 50 per cent of the costs related to back pain are incurred for chronic pain. The cause is often unknown. Much time may be spent looking for abnormalities such as a herniated disk, an annular tear, spinal stenosis, or spondylolisthesis, but these are seldom found; abnormalities detected on MRI scans are frequently unrelated to the symptoms. Factors which correlate with pain are cardiorespiratory disease, smoking, psychological morbidity, and adverse social conditions.

The association with smoking is probably due to atherosclerosis. There is now evidence that vascular damage is important in chronic backache. Degenerative disk disease is associated with atherosclerosis and spinal artery stenosis which leads to damage to the annulus fibrosus. Pressure on veins due to disk degeneration and protrusion leads to nerve root damage.

Sympathetically maintained pain is also important and recent work suggests that such pain may arise from altered central modulation within the spinal cord. Peripheral nerve injury increases the excitability of the central nervous system. The dorsal horn receptor fields may expand so that pain is felt over a much wider area than would be expected. Changes within the brain itself may also occur in back pain, with abnormal activation of the cingulate region. Similar changes are found in atypical facial pain, which helps to explain why there is a connection between physical and psychological factors in the causation of both kinds of pain. This suggests that, for many patients, chronic back pain is not the same as acute back pain lasting longer but is a different clinical entity (Jayson, 1997). It may also partly explain the effectiveness of acupuncture in chronic low back pain. Acupuncture, in other words, may act by modulating the way in which central pain mechanisms operate. Psychological and neurological influences are so closely interwoven in these circumstances that it becomes almost meaningless to ask whether the response is due to the 'placebo effect'.

Types of low back pain

There are several different types of low back pain, not all of which are suitable for acupuncture. It is important to take a full history and to carry out a physical examination before considering acupuncture.

1. Local back pain is due to compression or irritation of sensitive tissues; the causes include fractures, tears, or stretching of pain-sensitive tissues. This type of pain is accurately localized, often to the tips of the vertebral spines or the interspinous ligament. Acupuncture can be

useful in these cases. Pain that doesn't vary with changes in position may be due to tumour or infection. This is type B pain (Chapter 8).

2. Spinal origin pain (type A) is dull, diffuse, and aching in quality. It is poorly localized and its distribution does not correspond with that of a particular spinal segment. It may be felt in the spine itself or may radiate to the buttock, groin, anterior thigh, or anywhere down the leg, occasionally as far as the foot. The cause of this kind of pain is unknown. It is suitable for acupuncture treatment.

3. True radicular pain (type C) is different from the pain just discussed; it is sharp and 'electric' in quality and tends to follow a spinal segmental pattern. There may be areas of altered sensation and loss of reflexes. Coughing, sneezing, and straining at stool often make the pain worse. Changes in position that stretch the nerve roots may cause pain. If the sciatic nerve is affected (L5, S1), sitting may be painful and so may the straight leg raising test; if there is femoral nerve involvement (L2, L3, L4) sitting is not troublesome but the patient may be unable to straighten up. Since radicular pain is due to anatomical compression of nerve roots it isn't to be expected that acupuncture will be of much direct benefit in this case.

4. Muscle spasm is often cited as a cause of pain but the mechanism is unclear, and some people think that it isn't the spasm itself that is painful but rather the underlying lesion that is causing the spasm. The pain is dull in character and the patient's posture is altered by the spasm.

5. Pain may be referred to the spine from abdominal and pelvic viscera, but usually the pain is felt in the abdomen or pelvis as well as the back. Occasionally, however, it is confined to the back. It is often unaffected by position.

Acupuncture is worth considering for pain types 1, 2, and 4. It is unlikely to help in the others and is positively contraindicated in 5, because of its masking effect, unless a definite diagnosis has been made and the acupuncture is being applied as a palliative treatment, for example in malignancy.

Examining the back

It is essential to obtain a detailed history and carry out a full physical examination of the back when assessing a patient for the first time for possible acupuncture. The patient's gait and general demeanour may give important clues to the diagnosis. The spine should be considered as a whole, even though the symptoms may be confined to the lower back. Range of movement in all planes is checked, and it is customary to carry out the straight-leg raising test for sciatic tension, which is routinely taught to medical students, but this is probably the least useful

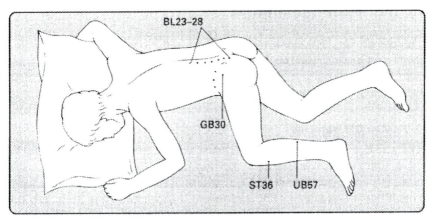

'Recovery position' for treating the back

examination in this region; a number of variants exist which are better. These include Lasègue's sign, in which the thigh is flexed to 90 degrees and then the knee is gradually extended, and the Bowstring test, which is similar to Lasègue's sign but with the addition of full dorsiflexion of the foot; pressure is then applied to the popliteal or posterior tibial nerve in the popliteal fossa. These tests are well described by Cummings, together with some others as well as a modification of his own (Cummings, 2000).

The history will often give a pointer to the possibility of referred pain; abdominal aneurysm should be excluded in middle-aged or elderly patients. The routine physical examination includes assessing the mobility of the hip and knee joints, neurological examination for sensation and reflexes, and verification of the pulses.

There are three possible positions in which one may place the patient to examine the back for trigger points and to carry out acupuncture: prone, sitting and leaning forwards, and the 'recovery position' – side lying, with the lowermost limb almost straight and the uppermost limb flexed. The degree of flexion in the hip must be adjusted to put the gluteal muscles under slight stretch but not excessive tension. The prone position, which might seem the most logical, is actually the least useful, because the paraspinal muscles are then completely relaxed whereas they should be under slight tension, and the vertebrae are squashed together. It is possible to reduce these disadvantages by placing one or two pillows under the patient's abdomen, but it is generally better to use one of the other positions for treatment. However, it is sometimes advisable first to examine the prone patient to search for local tenderness of individual vertebrae by pressing their spines, while the recovery position is needed if the gluteal region is to be needled.

Acupuncture techniques

The spinal cord terminates at the lower border of L1 in adults (actually, this is somewhat variable), and needling can therefore be carried out below this level fairly safely. The following ATAs are often used; as usual, they include both soft-tissue and periosteal sites.

1. Paraspinal muscles

The corresponding classic acupuncture points in this region are BL23–BL28, but I don't myself use this terminology; great precision is not required, nor have I found that it is essential to identify particular trigger points here. The needles are inserted to a depth of about 2 cm into the muscles. Deeper insertion will become periosteal acupuncture, described below.

2. Lumbar vertebrae

These are an important site for periosteal needling. The needle is inserted a little to one side of the midline and angled slightly inwards, so that its point comes to the side of the spinous process or to the lamina of the vertebra. It is possible to needle fairly vigorously in this region, since there is seldom much discomfort from the treatment. One or more vertebrae may be treated, usually bilaterally.

Some patients, especially older ones, have pain confined to the lower back ('saddle area'), and in these it is often enough to insert three or four needles into the paraspinal muscles in the region to a depth of about 2 or 3 cm. There is no need to try to needle specifically tender areas; treatment of the general area seems to work perfectly well, without trying to be exceedingly precise. Periosteal needling also seems to be unnecessary in these cases.

If one particular lumbar vertebra is noticeably tender, I generally carry out periosteal needling to that vertebra in the manner described above.

3. Sacroiliac region

This refers to the sacroiliac joint itself as well as to the ligaments connecting the sacrum and ilium (posterior sacroiliac, interosseus sacroiliac). The treatment may be done with the patient either sitting or lying, although sitting is easier. The visual landmark is the posterior superior iliac spine, identified by a dimple, which overlies the centre of the sacroiliac joint. However, I generally prefer to rely on the sense of touch. The palpating finger or thumb is drawn medially across the posterior iliac spine and then falls into the groove between the sacrum and the ilium; sometimes firm pressure is needed to identify this gap. The needle (usually 50 mm) is inserted through the skin and is angled slightly outwards so as to reach the sacroiliac joint. Needling this site commonly

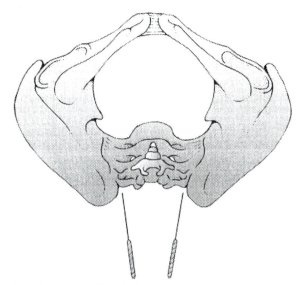

Needling sites for sacroiliac joints

causes referred sensation down the leg as far as the knee, and sometimes farther. The exact path taken by these sensations, and their character, are variable.

4. Quadratus lumborum

This muscle often seems to be neglected in acupuncture but it is a useful ATA, especially for the treatment of back pain in athletic people who play sports or who are ballet dancers. It is an approximately quadrilateral muscle, which arises from the iliolumbar ligament and the adjacent iliac crest for about 5 cm and is inserted into the medial half of the last rib and also into the tips of the transverse processes of the upper four lumbar vertebrae. To palpate it, press downwards and medially, above the crest of the ilium and towards the upper surface of the sacrum. Needling is done in the same direction, with the patient lying on the side and supported by one or two cushions under the lumbar vertebrae to stop the spine from sagging.

5. Gluteal muscles and the piriformis syndrome

These muscles commonly contain triggers in patients who have pain in the gluteal region or radiating down the lower limb. Although any of the gluteal muscles may be involved, one of the principal contenders for attention is piriformis, which is in close relation with both the sacroiliac joint and the sciatic nerve and lies almost parallel with the posterior margin of gluteus medius. It arises mainly from the front of the sacrum and passes out of the pelvis through the greater sciatic foramen and is inserted by a rounded tendon into the greater trochanter of the femur. In some people part or even all of the sciatic nerve pierces the piriformis and this arrangement has been thought to cause nerve entrapment. This is the usual explanation offered for the 'piriformis syndrome', though this may also be produced by trigger points within the muscle itself which could have the same consequence. This somewhat uncertain clinical entity has been well discussed by Cummings (2000), who acknowledges that it remains 'a controversial and esoteric clinical diagnosis'. Estimates of the frequency of the syndrome in patients with symptoms vary from 6 to 44 per cent. For the reasons discussed in Chapter 6, I am not convinced that the diagnostic concept of the piriformis syndrome is very useful.

In practice, I find that some patients have trigger points that appear to be in piriformis, while in others the maximum tenderness is apparently in gluteus medius or gluteus minimus. In any case, the acupuncture treatment consists in deep needling as accurately as possible into the site of tenderness. There is a classic acupuncture point in this area (GB30), generally said to lie one-third of the way along a line drawn from the highest point of the greater trochanter of the femur to the sacral hiatus. (This, of course, is a modern anatomical way of specifying its location; the traditional way is in terms of *cun*.) However, tenderness is the guiding feature of where to needle. Tenderness should be sought by means of progressively deeper palpation through gluteus maximus, which overlies it; this palpation may need to be fairly vigorous. (Note that the piriformis muscle cannot be palpated directly except via the rectum or vagina.)

To examine the region and to carry out the treatment the patient is placed in the 'recovery position' as already mentioned. It's important to get the amount of tension in the gluteal muscles right; too little and the trigger points won't be felt, too much and they will be obscured by the tautness of the muscles. We therefore adjust the degree of hip flexion as necessary. In patients with wide hips, it helps to place a pillow under the uppermost knee to prevent too much adduction of the thigh.

Triggers in this region are treated as a rule with deep needling (50 mm needle or longer). Students are often concerned about the possibility of damaging the sciatic nerve. However, the atraumatic tip of an acupuncture needle is fairly unlikely to do this, and moreover most damage to the sciatic nerve results from injection of fluids of various kinds. Nevertheless, direct insertion of the needle into the sciatic nerve should be avoided; piriformis lies above the point at which the nerve emerges from the greater sciatic foramen.

Strong de qi is often obtained in the gluteal region and the needle may be gripped so firmly that it cannot be withdrawn for some time. If this happen it should be left alone for a few minutes, until the spasm wears off. Books recommend inserting a second needle a short distance away from the trapped needle to release it, but this is seldom necessary in practice.

Success rates are generally quite high (about 70 per cent): patients who fail to respond are quite frequently those who eventually require surgery for persisting pain, due for example to prolapsed intervertebral disks.

In some male patients triggers in the lower back or gluteal region may refer pain to the scrotum. This at times leads to mistaken diagnoses of epididymitis, but needling of the relevant areas relieves the pain.

6. Greater trochanter of femur

This periosteal needling site is used for ostearthritic pain in the hip. It often provides good relief for 8–12 weeks after each treatment. The patient lies on the side with the affected hip uppermost, and either a 30 mm or a 50 mm needle is used to peck the periosteum, which may be done fairly vigorously at two or three sites. A fairly strong (0.30 mm diameter) needle is required.

Danger signs in back pain

The following clinical features suggest the possibility of serious pathology such as acute disk prolapse with neurological deficit, spinal fracture, spinal tumour or infection, and the cauda equina syndrome.

- Possible fracture
    History of major trauma, or minor trauma (even strenuous lifting) in older or potentially osteoporotic patient
- Possible tumour or infection
    Age over 50 or under 20
    Constitutional symptoms (fever, chills, weight loss)
    Risk factors for spinal infection (recent infection, IV drug abuse, immune suppression, diabetes)
    Pain worse when supine or severe night-time pain
- Possible cauda equina syndrome
    Saddle anaesthesia
    Recent onset of bladder dysfunction
    Severe or progressive neurological deficiency in lower limbs
    Laxity of anal sphincter
    Perianal or perineal sensory loss
    Major motor weakness

Surface anatomy

1. The spine of T3 is opposite the root of the scapular spine.
2. The spine of T7 is opposite the inferior angle of the scapula.
3. The eighth rib is just below the inferior angle of the scapula.

4. The spine of T12 is opposite the midpoint of a line drawn from the inferior angle of the scapula to the iliac crest.
5. A line joining the posterior iliac spines passes through the spine of S2.
6. The posterior superior iliac spine overlies the centre of the sacroiliac joint.
7. The lower limit of the spinal cord is at the interval between L1 and L2 in adults. This is just above the level of the elbow joint when the subject is standing with the arms beside the body. The subarachnoid space reaches the upper border of the third sacral spine.
8. The cervical pleura and lung reach the level of the spine of C7. They are represented by a convex line drawn from the sternoclavicular joint to the junction of the middle and medial thirds of the clavicle; the summit of this line is 3.5 cm above the clavicle.
9. The lower limit of the pleural sac reaches a point 2 cm lateral to the upper border of the spine of T12 and is indicated by a line drawn downwards and laterally from here to cut the lateral border of the sacrospinalis just where the tip of the twelfth rib emerges.
10. The kidneys are mapped by Morris's parallelogram: draw horizontal lines through the spines of T11 and L3, and vertical lines 2.5 and 9.5 cm from the median plane.

References

Cummings M. (2000) Piriformis syndrome. *Acupuncture in Medicine*, 18; 108–21.
Jayson M.I.V. (1997) Why does acute back pain become chronic? *British Medical Journal*, 314; 1639–40.

Chapter 13

The lower limb

In the lower limb we have a considerable number of ATAs, most of which are concerned with painful disorders in the region. However, there are also some (the 'spleen' points in the traditional system) that are supposed to be connected with the pelvic organs in women and which seem to be effective in certain gynaecological disorders.

The knee

Pain in the knee may be referred from the hip, which should therefore always be checked. There are also ATAs in the thigh that may refer pain to the knee.

Medial thigh area

There is a latent trigger at the medial side of the thigh, at the junction of the middle and lower thirds. This may cause knee pain, but I think only in young patients (below the age of about 21). It seems to be in vastus medialis. Needling this site gives relief in patients in this age group but not, in my experience, in older patients.

Posterior thigh area

There are latent trigger points at the back of the thigh (hamstrings), usually just lateral to the tendons of semimembranosus and semi-tendinosus. These trigger points may be activated by sitting for long periods on a hard chair, the edge of which presses on the tendons. The pain is referred to the front of the thigh, just above the patella. The history suggests the diagnosis.

Medial tibial platform

I use this admittedly unorthodox anatomical term to refer to an ATA consisting of the flattish area of bone below the knee joint; it is where the tibia is most superficial. In postmenopausal women, especially if they are overweight, there may be an oedematous swelling here, which is noticeably tender. Men and younger women may also be tender in this area but usually without the swelling. The whole region may be tender or only localized areas within it. This site is approximately SP9 in the traditional system, although most charts place SP9 rather farther posteriorly, in the muscles rather than over the bone.

This ATA is the main site for treating the knee and is often effective. Some sources advise carefully palpating the tissues round the knee for tender areas and needling those preferentially, but I am not convinced that this really makes much difference to the success rate; simply needling the periosteum anywhere in this region seems to be equally effective, whether or not it is tender. (Most periosteal acupuncture has this nonspecific character.) Some patients find the treatment painful, while others appear hardly to feel it.

Needling this ATA works for osteoarthritic knee pain among other causes, though, as usual, the more severe the disease the worse the results. However, I have seen good pain relief even when there is gross osteoarthritis. The treatment is therefore always worth trying. The usual duration of relief is about 12 weeks.

The patella

Some patients have knee pain that appears to be located behind the patella. In these cases I have needled the outer surface of the patella in two places, which seems to help; however, the treatment is painful so I don't use it routinely. It doesn't usually seem to help in the rather obscure disorder labelled chondromalacia of the patella.

Iliotibial band (tract) syndrome

This is typically a sports-related disorder. The iliotibial band or tract is a thickened part of the fascia lata, which is attached to all the prominent points around the knee (condyles of the femur and tibia, and head of the fibula). The tensor fasciae latae muscle is inserted between the two layers of the iliotibial tract and tightens the fascia lata, as its name implies. It helps in extension of the knee, and also in abduction and medial rotation of the thigh. In the erect posture it helps to steady the pelvis on the head of the femur; through the iliotibial tract it steadies the condyles of the femur on the tibia and thus helps to maintain the erect attitude.

As this description indicates, the tensor fasciae latae and the iliotibial band are important in activities such as running and walking. Physiotherapists find these structures important to treat in people such as footballers, cricketers, and ballet dancers. They knead the lateral surface of the thigh with their knuckles to detect triggers in the muscle and needle those.

It is also possible to develop a trigger in the iliotibial tract as it passes beside the knee.

> Some years ago, while on a cycling tour in Greece, I found I was suffering a lot of knee pain on about the second day. This followed a day's walking on rough ground at the site of the temple at Delphi. As I was planning to do a long ride the next day (160 kilometres – 100 miles – with four passes of about 1500 metres) this was a serious matter and I wondered whether I should consider abandoning the tour. The pain was felt over the whole anterior surface of the knee, but when I examined the joint I found a markedly tender area at the lateral side of the knee over the iliotibial tract. I therefore needled this fairly superficially, to avoid going into the knee joint. By next morning the pain was a lot less and I completed the day's ride without incident; by the time I arrived at my destination there was no pain at all. There was a slight recurrence of pain after about 10 days; I sat down beside the road and repeated the treatment, and have never had any pain of that kind subsequently.

Leg muscles

There are a number of ATAs in the muscles of the leg, including some which are also named acupuncture points in the traditional system.

SP6: This is a classic acupuncture point, in the soleus muscle on the medial side of the leg above the ankle. It is commonly tender in both sexes and is thus a latent trigger point. In the classic system it is related to gynaecological disorders of all kinds, and this is probably a real effect. Needling this site is an effective treatment of dysmenorrhoea, and may sometimes help in menorrhagia and similar functional disorders, though I am less certain of this. SP9, a site in the leg muscles just below the knee on the medial side, and SP10, above the knee, are used similarly. These spleen points are among the 'forbidden areas' in pregnancy; others are the lower abdomen and the lower back. SP6 has on occasion been used to induce labour, and sometimes seems to be effective for this purpose, though there is no good supporting evidence.

Other named acupuncture points in this region include BL57 on the back of the leg, between the bellies of the gastrocnemius muscle, and ST36, in the peroneal muscles below the knee. However, I am not convinced that it is necessary to needle these sites specifically, and in many cases needling anywhere in the muscles of the leg ('random needling') appears to be effective. I generally treat about six points here, three on each side of the leg.

Random needling of the leg can be used to treat pain in the leg from a variety of causes, especially vascular pain due to arterial insufficiency. It also helps some patients with pain due to diabetic neuropathy. Some patients with restless legs also respond.

> A man in his 70s had been unable to sleep for some years owing to severe night-time pain. He had arteriosclerotic narrowing of his arteries and had had surgery for this, which had not relieved his pain. Needling his legs allowed him to sleep without pain; the treatment was repeated every three months for several years until his death.

Triggers in the leg muscles may cause radiation of pain to the sole of the foot. This is often labelled 'plantar fasciitis', although there seems to be little evidence that this is really a fasciitis. Needling the muscles sometimes gives relief. More often, however, treatment is needed to the sole itself (see below).

Phantom limb pain

Patients who have had limbs amputated for any reason may experience pain in the absent limb. Acupuncture textbooks often recommend treating the opposite limb in such cases, but I have had more success when I have needled the stump of the amputated limb.

> A woman in her 70s who had had an above-knee amputation for arterial disease was experiencing a lot of pain at night, which prevented her from sleeping. Acupuncture to the stump allowed her to sleep but the treatment needed to be done frequently; I therefore taught the companion she lived with to do it and this afforded her good relief.

The sole

Many patients suffer from pain in the sole which is usually ascribed to plantar fasciitis. The theory is that repeated trauma to the plantar fascia causes damage to the attachment to the calcaneum, which gives rise to pain. If the foot is X-rayed a calcaneal bony spur may be found and this is often alleged to be the cause of the pain; however, it's unclear that the incidence of spurs in patients with pain in the sole is greater than in the general population.

In some cases pain in the sole appears to be due to trigger points in the gastrocnemius muscle, and it is always worth looking here first because treatment of these ATAs is relatively painless. However, in many cases this approach is unsuccessful and then the treatment is to needle the calcaneum itself through the sole. There are generally one or two painful areas, usually situated at the anterior end of the calcaneum. These are identified by firm palpation, and a needle may then be inserted through the sole to the periosteum, which is pecked. This is inevitably a painful treatment and patients must be warned of this before it is done; however, the pain from their disorder is generally so severe that they are prepared to try almost anything, and the treatment is often successful, although two or three sessions may be required to get full relief.

Pain in the ankle: it's relatively unusual for this joint to be affected by osteoarthritis, which is perhaps surprising in view of its weight-bearing role. However, if it becomes painful it can be treated in the usual way, by periosteal pecking; this may be done to the distal end of the tibia, above the joint margin, and to the navicular.

Achilles tendonitis can be treated by surrounding the swelling with short needles. This helps the pain although it makes little difference to the swelling. The needles should not be inserted into the tendon.

Pain in the big toe (first carpometacarpal joint): generally due to osteoarthritis. This responds exceptionally well to treatment. Four sites are needled, over the shaft of the bones above and below the joint, thus avoiding the tendon in the midline. Relief after each treatment generally lasts for 12 weeks.

Pain in the forefoot (metatarsalgia): I have not treated this frequently myself but a podietrist has reported good results using needling of the interosseous muscles. Needling the interosseous muscles seems to be less effective here than in the hand.

The classic acupuncture point LR3 is situated in the middle of the interspace between the first and second metatarsal bones (its exact location is shown slightly variably in different sources). I regard this as one of the major 'general stimulation sites' and I therefore discuss it separately in that context in Chapter 15.

Chapter 14

The abdomen

Needling the anterior abdominal wall is, in my experience, a very effective acupuncture technique, but it is difficult to explain why it should work. I initially thought of treating this area after reading about it in the Travell & Simons (1983) manual. These authors identify trigger points in the abdominal wall, which they say are responsible not only for pain but also for symptoms such as chronic diarrhoea. Their identification of these sites as trigger points is in keeping with their general approach, but I have not been able to convince myself that this is really the basis of the treatment. When needling this area I don't search for tender areas specifically but the acupuncture is nevertheless effective, and I therefore describe my treatment as based on ATAs rather than on trigger points.

As a rule, I find that needling below the umbilicus is more effective than needling above it. I have on occasion tried to treat non-ulcer dyspepsia by needling the epigastrium but the results have been unconvincing. My most notable success with treating this area occurred in a young man who had been hiccupping for 24 hours; a single needle in his epigastrium stopped the hiccups at once, but I have not had an opportunity to try this treatment again.

The lower abdomen, below the umbilicus, is a fruitful acupuncture area. There are named acupuncture points in this region (SP13–15, ST25–28, K12–16, CV3–8), but I do not use these terms and simply regard the whole area as a large ATA. Treatment consists in subcutaneous needling; I usually put in two rows of needles below the umbilicus, giving a total of 8–12, depending on the size of the patient. If one area of the abdomen is notably tender or painful, I put more needles in there, though I am not sure that this is essential. Short (15 mm) needles are adequate, and provide a safety net to prevent entering the abdominal cavity if the patient is thin. (In a very thin patient the needles should, as usual, be inserted at an angle.)

Acupuncture books often advise needling the corresponding areas of the back for abdominal problems (BL22–25, BL46–47), but I haven't found that using these improves the results, nor have I found any additional effect from using distant points such as ST36, which is also recommended, and I therefore seldom do more than treat the abdomen in the manner described, although I sometimes add LR3 as a generalized stimulation point.

This treatment can be useful in a wide range of abdominal disorders, especially those characterized by pain: for example, diverticular disease.

A middle-aged man came for treatment of his diverticular disease. This was of great severity; he was in constant pain and had had to take early retirement in consequence. This was fairly early in my acupuncture career and I had no experience of treating such symptoms with acupuncture, so my suggestion of putting in some needles was made hesitantly. The patient accepted, and I put in some needles in LR3 and also in his abdomen. Almost at once he appeared to go into a kind of trance; he felt totally ecstatic. He turned out, in fact, to be one of the strongest reactors I ever encountered. After this initial treatment he had no pain at all for 6 weeks. After a few more sessions the duration of relief had increased to 12 weeks, and he continued to feel ecstatic each time the needles were inserted. Eventually I taught him to do the treatment himself, and this appeared to work equally well.

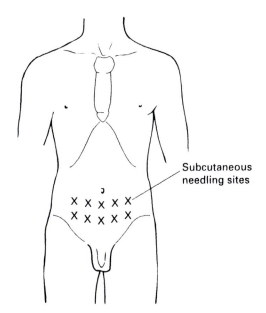

Needling sites in lower abdomen

Abdominal wall needling also often works for unexplained abdominal pain. This is of course a worrying symptom, and some patients with unexplained pain later go on to be diagnosed with serious diseases such as carcinoma of the colon, but there is certainly a group who do not have an identifiable disease. In cases where serious abdominal pathology has been definitely excluded, therefore, acupuncture is certainly worth trying.

Nowadays there is a tendency to label all unexplained abdominal symptoms as 'irritable bowel'. This is a mistake; the term should be restricted to the classic clinical picture of alternating constipation and diarrhoea, bloating, and pain. So far as acupuncture is concerned in irritable bowel, treatment is often effective for pain but less so for other symptoms.

Perhaps the most surprising success with acupuncture that I have encountered is in the treatment of ulcerative colitis. I first tried this many years ago, in a patient whom I was treating for something else. One day she chanced to mention that she also suffered from colitis and asked if acupuncture would help. I said that I thought it might help the pain if she was lucky but would have no effect on the bleeding or diarrhoea. She nevertheless asked me to try, and I therefore needled her lower abdomen in the manner just described. To my surprise, she came back a couple of weeks later to report that all her symptoms, not just the pain, were improved. I therefore continued to treat her and within a few visits she had gone into remission.

Encouraged by this, I tried the treatment out on some further patients, and the results were surprisingly good. One woman said she always had a sudden urgent bowel motion about half an hour after acupuncture, after which she was symptom-free for many months. Another patient was a young girl, aged 11 when I started treatment; both her mother and her grandmother had the same disease. Acupuncture produced an almost complete remission in her case. A colleague and I at my hospital used acupuncture to treat some 30 patients with ulcerative colitis during the time I was there. At least three-quarters of those treated had a worthwhile improvement, and some apparently went into complete remission.

We saw fewer patients with Crohn's disease than with ulcerative colitis, so it is difficult to be certain of the effectiveness of acupuncture for this disorder, but we had the impression that it didn't work so well here. This is surprising in one way, because the two diseases have quite similar symptoms, but not in another, because they are different pathologically.

The lower abdomen can be needled in gynaecological disorders, such as dysmenorrhoea or pelvic inflammatory disease, although the ATA on the medial side of the leg (SP6) should be treated as well in these cases. There have been reports that needling the abdomen helps in bladder disorders such as unstable bladder, but I have not seen enough of these cases to be confident of its effectiveness.

Painful scars

I will discuss the treatment of these here, since painful postoperative scars often occur in the abdomen; however scars in any part of the body may be treated in a similar way, and the results are nearly always excellent. This applies both to postoperative and to traumatic scars.

The treatment is, as usual, very simple. One possibility is to needle around the scar, but this doesn't always work. In most cases it is necessary to insert the needle directly into the scar itself, choosing the sites of maximum tenderness. Quite a number of needles may be required, depending on the length of the scar. Sometimes one treatment is enough.

> A man had had pain in an abdominal scar following surgery some 20 years previously. A few needles were inserted; the pain disappeared immediately and never returned.

Instant cures such as this are of course gratifying as well as surprising, but more often several sessions are necessary.

> A woman had surgery to her foot for metatarsalgia. She was left with a painful scar in the sole between the first and second toes, so that she found walking difficult. The scar was about an inch long (2.5 cm) and the distal part was red and angry-looking. Initially I treated this by needling around the scar, but when this failed I told her that the only choice was to needle the scar itself, which would hurt. She agreed to this, so I needled the reddened part of the scar. Within two or three sessions the redness had vanished and so had the pain; there was no recurrence after three years.

(Incidentally, P.D. Wall says that although this operation is supposed to work by removing a neuroma, in most cases no nerve tissue is found in the material if it is examined histologically, which suggests that the operation must produce its effects in some other way (Wall, 1999). This is just one of the many puzzling features of pain.)

References

Travell J.G. & Simons D.G. (1983) *Myofascial Pain and Dysfunction. The trigger point manual*. Vol. 1. Williams & Wilkins, Baltimore.
Wall P. (1999) *Pain: the science of suffering*. Weidenfeld & Nicolson, London.

Chapter 15

Generalized stimulation

Quite a few doctors who take up acupuncture seem to have a mental block about using it for anything other than the relief of musculoskeletal pain. There are probably two main reasons for this attitude. One is a feeling that there is some respectable scientific basis for the use of needles to relieve this kind of pain, probably on the basis of counter-irritation, but little or none to support the treatment of non-painful disorders.

There is some truth in this, although the use of PC6 to treat nausea and vomiting has received probably more attention from Western researchers than any other acupuncture procedure, and this is not concerned with pain. But there are reasonably plausible neurological explanations for how acupuncture might relieve pain, whereas there is little to explain how it might work in other circumstances. Nevertheless, it has to be admitted that, even for pain, most of the evidence for the effectiveness of acupuncture is anecdotal, so the acupuncture treatment of non-painful disorders is not in much worse case than the treatment of pain.

The other reason for doctors' reluctance to embark on using acupuncture to treat non-painful disorders is a vague awareness that it depends on using traditional acupuncture which is a highly esoteric business, requiring the therapist to select complicated combinations of points on an individual basis, and presupposing an acceptance of unfamiliar alien ideas. Advocates of the traditional system would, naturally, endorse such views.

My position is (as you might expect by now) somewhat different. My experience indicates that, although acupuncture is certainly no sort of panacea, it does work for certain disorders not characterised by pain. I don't, however, accept the traditional ideas about the specificity of individual acupuncture points, nor do I think that elaborate forms of treatment are necessary in treating these rather heterogeneous clinical problems. This does not involve any kind of 'advanced acupuncture', and indeed in most cases the treatment is very simple, because all that is required is general stimulation. In other words, it is a nonspecific effect, that can in principle be produced by needling anywhere in the body. However, certain areas, notably the hands and feet, seem to be the most effective sites. I find that needling the feet is more effective than the hands, and probably less painful. LI4, in the hand, is often used, but it can be painful, and it seems occasionally to cause adverse reactions. As mentioned in Chapter 4, I have seen one case, in which it was used as a practice site on an acupuncture course, where the doctor concerned had pain in the thumb for six months afterwards, and there has recently been a report of bilateral hand oedema, lasting for several weeks, after it was used to treat back pain (McCartney *et al.*, 2000). Another popular point is ST36, located in the tibialis anterior muscle, below the knee. This is claimed by some to be capable of stimulating the immune system.

Although I needle both the above sites from time to time, I agree with Mann that the classic acupuncture point LR3 is generally the best site to use. However, I'm also sure he is right in saying that, in many people, anywhere on the dorsum of the foot, or even a larger area, might be equally effective.

LR3 is situated between the first and second metatarsal bones. It is normally needled to a depth of about 0.5 in (12 mm). Different books show slightly variable locations for the point but this is unimportant. The target area is a roughly rectangular area about an inch (2.5 cm) long and a quarter of an inch (0.6 cm) wide, situated between the first and second metatarsal bones. It tapers to a point proximally, where the two metatarsal bones abut each other; below, it ends in the web of skin between the toes. It is occupied by muscles (the dorsal and plantar interossei) and contains the dorsalis pedis artery and one of its branches, the first dorsal metatarsal artery; on its fibular side the dorsalis pedis artery is related to the medial terminal branch of the anterior tibial nerve. Theoretically these structures might be damaged when needling in this region but in practice this very seldom occurs. However, some oozing of blood may be seen when the patient stands up, owing to increased hydrostatic pressure. (Note that the dorsalis pedis artery is somewhat variable: it may be larger than normal or absent, and it frequently curves laterally.)

LR3 and similar points can be used to treat a wide range of disorders, either as a complete treatment or as an adjunct to local needling. Needling LR3 is particularly likely to cause the euphoria and other subjective effects that characterize a strong reactor.

It's difficult to give a complete list of disorders and symptoms that may be treated by generalized stimulation, partly because a lot depends on the reactivity of the individual patient. If someone is a good acupuncture subject it may be possible to obtain surprisingly good results in such a person, even in unpromising disorders.

Here is a brief description of the disorders that I have principally used generalized stimulation for.

A woman in her 40s came for treatment of a mysterious syndrome. Throughout the summer she suffered a skin rash whenever she went out in the sun, so that she had to remain indoors. Throughout the winter she had diarrhoea with bleeding; she had been investigated by gastroenterologists without any cause being identified. A few treatments to LR3 produced a complete remission in both sets of symptoms; the effect lasted at least a year, after which I didn't see her again.

Solar dermatitis

The case report above reflects a more general trend, which is that solar dermatitis appears to respond particularly well to acupuncture. The converse may, I think, also be true: patients who suffer from solar dermatitis may be good acupuncture subjects.

Chronic urticaria

This is, presumably, an allergic disorder, although it is seldom possible to identify the offending foodstuff or other agent responsible. Acupuncture often helps with the symptoms but the effects of treatment are generally short-lived, so that it is one of the disorders where patients may need to treat themselves. Some patients report that, after acupuncture, they are now able to eat foods which formerly they couldn't tolerate. I am quite prepared to accept that this may be, at least in part, the result of self-suggestion, but it's nevertheless valuable.

Menopausal hot flushes

Menopausal flushes often respond to acupuncture, although, again, the effect may be brief, so that self-acupuncture is indicated. Men suffering from flushes as a result of hormonal treatment for prostate cancer also respond.

Bronchial asthma

Randomized controlled trials of acupuncture in asthma have generally not shown any effect, and I would agree with this; most patients I have tried it on have not responded. There is, however, a small number in whom it is dramatically effective, with immediate increases in peak flow of up to 400 per cent. Cookbooks recommend a number of points on the chest and elsewhere for asthma, but having tried them I am not impressed. I now think that if anything is going to work, it is LR3; if that doesn't work, you may as well forget using acupuncture.

A young woman, whom I already knew to be a strong reactor to acupuncture, came to the hospital outpatient department in a severe asthmatic attack. She was wheezing loudly and her peak flow rate was 110 litres per minute. I said that I didn't think acupuncture was going to work, but I would do it anyway. I put a needle in LR3; she immediately felt much better and her peak flow rate was now 440 L/min. I said that this was fine but it was unlikely to last and she should go to her doctor next day for some prednisolone. (She lived a long way from London so couldn't attend for further treatment very easily.) However, she returned six weeks later, still feeling well, and her peak flow rate was still 440 L/min.

A middle-aged woman who had suffered severely from asthma for many years came for treatment. She had been admitted to hospital with asthma on several occasions and had constant symptoms in spite of treatment. She had a stressful job which was no doubt making matters worse. When she came to see me her peak flow rate was 110 L/min. I tried acupuncture at LR3: immediately her peak flow went up to 440 L/min. Like the previous patient, she lived a long way from London. I asked her to keep a record of her peak flow readings at home. When she returned some six weeks later, the readings showed that her peak flow had remained high for several weeks after treatment but had gradually reverted to its previous low level. After she had attended for more treatments over about a year, I taught her to needle herself at LR3. She continued to remain well provided she did this, and required no further hospital admissions.

Hay fever asthma often does well.

A woman in her 40s had asthma only in summer; it was pollen-related. Over several years I treated her a couple of times at LR3 in early May; provided this was done she had no asthma during the summer, but one year when she failed to attend for treatment she had bad asthma again all summer.

Probably only about 10 per cent of patients with asthma, possibly fewer, will respond, but in some of those, as indicated by these case reports, acupuncture is extremely effective. However, it's important to verify the effect of the treatment by means of peak flow studies.

preferably done at home over several weeks, since subjective impressions of improvement are sometimes misleading.

It's not easy to predict which patients will do well. Acupuncture is probably most likely to work in patients who are strongly allergic, but this is not invariably the case.

Remember the possibility of aggravation, which may lead to an episode of status asthmaticus if an asthmatic person is treated too strongly. However, this is very unlikely to happen with the kind of treatment described in this book.

Headache and migraine

As described in Chapter 9, some patients respond better to LR3 than to local acupuncture directed to the head and neck. I would normally try both forms of treatment in a case of migraine before giving up. Occasionally, however, treating LR3 appears to produce only an aggravation, without subsequent improvement.

A middle-aged woman came for treatment of her migraine. I tried LR3, and within half an hour she had a migraine of exceptional severity, preceded by a visual aura (the first she had ever experienced). On the second occasion I repeated the acupuncture, on one side only, with minimal stimulation. The result was the same: a severe migraine within half an hour. However, I felt that I must be on the right track since at least I was having some effect, and the general principle in acupuncture is that if you can make symptoms worse with your treatment you can probably also make them better. So on her third attendance I needled LR3 as lightly as I could, just breaking the skin. Once more she experienced a severe migraine, at which point we agreed jointly to give up.

Migraine equivalents

These are focal neurological symptoms that occur without headaches or vomiting and are most frequent in patients between the ages of 40 and 70, in whom they may occur after the headaches have ceased. In children, benign paroxysmal vertigo and episodic abdominal pain are other manifestations of this syndrome. I have a personal interest in this because, as a teenager and into my early 20s, I used to suffer what I now realize were migraine equivalents. In these I would feel as if reality were subtly altered in some indescribable way. The state would last for about 20 minutes and then pass off, without a subsequent headache, although I did have classic migraines at other times.

Migraine equivalents can be of almost any character and I suspect are probably more common than is sometimes recognized. Acupuncture at LR3 is worth trying in any case of transient neurological disturbance in which serious organic disease has been excluded.

Reference

McCartney C.J.L., Herriot R. & Chambers W.A. (2000). Bilateral hand oedema related to acupuncture. *Pain*, 84: 429–30.

Part 4

Chapter 16

Electricity in acupuncture

Electricity has been used in two main ways in acupuncture: for needle stimulation and for 'point detection'. Transcutaneous electrical nerve stimulation (TENS) is a method of pain relief that uses electricity, and although it is not acupuncture it is often discussed in the same context. A more recent application of electricity to acupuncture is the use of low-power lasers in place of needles.

Needle stimulation by electricity (White, 1998)

The application of electricity to needles is a Chinese innovation. The technique was originally used as an adjunct to acupuncture analgesia for surgery, which had begun in the 1950s with the encouragement of Chairman Mao. At first, anaesthetists manipulated the needles manually while the surgical operation was being performed, but this was tedious and so electrical pulse generators were introduced as a substitute. It is now clear that the effectiveness and scope of acupuncture analgesia were considerably exaggerated in China, and some Western commentators (for example, see Wall, 1999), think that it can be attributed to hypnotism. Electrical stimulation, however, was taken up in the West and was used quite widely in the treatment of pain.

Clinically, electrical stimulation of needles is usually done by attaching crocodile clips; obviously at least two needles must be inserted in order to complete the circuit and often several pairs of needles are used. Direct current is unsuitable because it causes an electrochemical effect which weakens the needles and ultimately causes them to break. The same applies to a monophasic wave, so a biphasic pulsed wave is used. The electrical parameters are the voltage (up to 20 V), the current (10–50 mA), the wave form (square wave), the pulse width (0.05–0.5 ms), the polarity (biphasic, as already noted), and the frequency range (anywhere between less than 10 Hz and more than 100 Hz). There is some evidence that low-frequency stimulation is more effective than high-frequency stimulation. Many machines allow for automatically varying the frequency so as to try to reduce habituation to the stimulus.

The patient must feel the current but it should not be painful. The dangers of the procedure are the same as those for manual acupuncture, but in addition it is contraindicated if the patient has a demand pacemaker.

There are few clinical trials comparing electrical and manual acupuncture and so, in the absence of definite information, the choice of which to use comes down largely to personal preference. When I first started using acupuncture I tried applying electrical stimulation in inpatients with a fair amount of success, but I was not convinced that the results were any better than those achieved with brief manual stimulation. I now think that the electrical approach has little to offer, and for the sort of brief stimulation that I advocate it would clearly be irrelevant. It would be going too far to say that electrical stimulation can never offer any advantage, but in the vast majority of cases manual stimulation is equally and possibly more effective, and much simpler to apply.

Transcutaneous electrical nerve stimulation
(Thompson, 1998)

TENS is similar to electro-acupuncture in a number of ways, the principal difference being that the electricity is transmitted through the skin via conducting pads instead of via needles. Another difference is that low-intensity, high-frequency stimulation is most commonly used (40–150 Hz, 10–30 mA). However, some machines offer a 'burst' facility, with interrupted trains of fast (100 Hz) stimulation to give an effective pulse frequency which may be as low as 2 Hz; this causes tetanic twitching in the stimulated muscles. Because habituation occurs with

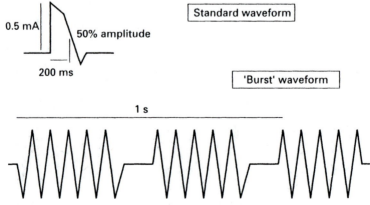

Electrical waveform characteristics of TENS

TENS, as it does with electrical stimulation of needles, there have been attempts to design more sophisticated machines to vary the pulse pattern either rhythmically or randomly.

The TENS apparatus consists essentially of the stimulator, which is battery-operated and is about the size of a cigarette packet, together with the connecting leads and the electrodes or pads. The minimum controls are one to regulate the amplitude of the current and another to regulate the frequency. Some machines allow the pulse width (the duration of each pulse) to be altered but in most it is fixed. Many manufacturers now produce TENS machines and patients can buy them by mail order quite easily.

It is important to make sure that patients give TENS a proper trial and understand clearly how to use the machine. They must be able to feel the stimulation, which causes a tingling sensation. The nervous system adapts quickly to the stimulus and therefore the amplitude of the current has to be increased after a few minutes' use. Initially patients should use the machine for at least an hour three times a day; alternatively, they can use it all day. Pain relief generally occurs soon after the machine is switched on; if it doesn't, the position of the electrodes or the setting of the controls should be altered. Trial and error are essential for success. Patients also need to understand that relief is often felt only while the stimulation is happening; if there is a carry-over into the post-stimulation time this is a bonus but it doesn't always occur.

TENS is generally safe, the main problem being skin irritation at the sites of the electrodes. This can be minimized by making sure that the area of skin to which the electrodes are applied is kept dry and free from grease and cosmetics; this applies both to the carbon rubber electrodes, which require electrode jelly, and the self-adhesive type. Like electro-acupuncture, TENS should not be used in patients with demand pacemakers. It should also not be applied to the front of the neck, to avoid the theoretical possibility of stimulating the nerves of the carotid sinus, causing hypotension, or the larynx, causing laryngeal spasm.

Choosing where to place the electrodes is important. The commonest method is to place them on either side of the painful area; another idea is to place them over a main nerve leading to the area. A third recommendation is to place them over the spinal cord, two or three segments above the painful segment, but this is less often effective.

TENS is used to treat both acute and chronic pain; success has also been claimed for its use in labour pain. TENS can relieve some kinds of pain that are otherwise difficult to treat: for example, neuropathic pain (post-herpetic neuralgia) and pain due to brachial plexus avulsion and spinal cord trauma. However, the response to TENS is not always sustained over time; this may be due to an increase in the pain level or to a change in the patient's response to TENS. The original response may have been a placebo effect, or tolerance to TENS may develop through various mechanisms.

The relation between acupuncture and TENS is somewhat complicated. Some patients will respond to acupuncture but not TENS; some will respond to TENS but not acupuncture; some will respond to both. It is often worth trying TENS in patients who do not improve with acupuncture or who do so for only short periods. In some painful disorders, such as post-herpetic neuralgia, TENS is much more likely to succeed than is acupuncture. The unpredictability of response must however always be kept in mind.

> A woman had had a lumbar puncture performed at another hospital. The procedure had been technically difficult, and in the process a nerve root in the cauda equina had been damaged, resulting in severe pain in the leg that persisted for many months. I thought she would respond to TENS so got her into hospital for an extended trial of this treatment. After a week she was no better. On the morning she was to be discharged I tried acupuncture at LR3 on the painful side, with no real expectation that it would help, but to my surprise it produced immediate relief. After a few more treatments at intervals she was practically pain-free.

Non-pain use of TENS

I have found that TENS will relieve spasm in some patients with multiple sclerosis. For example, if the electrodes are placed over the femoral nerve in a patient whose leg is in spasm, it may become flaccid immediately. This is not always desirable, since it can make it impossible for the patient to stand up; but it is at least of theoretical interest and can on occasion be useful in practice. However, it never seems to work in patients who have had a spinal cord transection due to trauma.

Lasers and acupuncture

The use of low-power lasers to stimulate acupuncture points began to be developed in the 1970s. The appeal of this idea is evident, since the treatment is pain-free and therefore suitable for children or people who are afraid of acupuncture; also, there is no risk of infection. However, many questions remain. Are lasers in any way comparable to acupuncture in their effects, and do they really do anything or is their effect entirely that of a powerful placebo? These questions have been addressed by Baldry (1998) in a review of the controlled studies then available, his conclusion being that the evidence so far does not favour this form of treatment. Other reviews have found the same lack of convincing effect. It is not only that most controlled trials have failed to show a genuine effect; it's also difficult to advance a scientific explanation for how a low-power laser could be thought to affect the tissues in the same way as an acupuncture needle.

There is quite good evidence that low-power lasers can accelerate healing of superficial lesions such as burns and ulcers. This effect is most pronounced at a frequency of 700 Hz and is inhibited at 1200 Hz. However, laser light is not required for this; non-coherent natural light seems to work equally well.

I conclude, from the available information, together with some personal testing of a laser a few years ago, that this form of treatment has little to offer the practising acupuncturist. Anyone who wishes to experiment with a laser needs to keep in mind that the use of such apparatus is regulated by law, because of the danger of causing retinal damage if the beam is directed at the eye.

'Point detection'

There are many machines on the market which purport to detect acupuncture points electrically; some also apply electrical stimulation as a form of treatment. Most depend on the theory that acupuncture points are areas of reduced skin resistance. The machines usually have a neutral electrode plus a searching electrode ending in a blunt point. The patient holds the neutral electrode and the operator moves the searching electrode about on the skin, looking for the sites of reduced resistance, which are signalled by a buzzer or a deflection on a pointer.

The weakness of nearly all these machines is that it is very easy to produce artifacts when using them. Leaving the probe a little longer in one place on the skin or pressing a little harder will produce an 'acupuncture point' almost anywhere. Some more sophisticated machines have been developed in an attempt to get round this difficulty but most have been used only in a research context. A study was carried out at Upstate Medical Center, Syracuse, New York (Reichmanis & Becker, 1976), in which the measuring electrode assembly consisted of 36 steel rods in a 6 × 6 square, connected to a dc Wheatstone bridge circuit. Using this rather elaborate apparatus the researchers were able to demonstrate local variations in conductance at a number of classic acupuncture points on the Triple Energizer and Lung channels, although not all the points were detected in every subject.

A few years earlier, Brown and colleagues (1974) at the University of Missouri School of Medicine used a device that did not apply a current to the skin but instead measured the electrical activity of the body itself. The outer surface of the skin is electrically negative with respect to subcutaneous tissue, and the experimenters used this fact to test for acupuncture points. They found 18 points on the upper arm, which included all those shown as acupuncture points on charts as well as a few not shown. These points were distributed symmetrically on the two arms and did not change in situation or electrical activity over time.

At a more practical level, the most useful machine for detecting local electrical differences in the skin seems to be a Japanese device called the Neurometer, which is used for a neoclassic form of acupuncture in Japan called Ryodoraku. This machine puts out a brief spike of current every 0.6 seconds and measures the resistance to this. Needham and Gwei-Djen (1980) report a convincing demonstration of many acupuncture points with the Neurometer; moreover these points could still be demonstrated on a cadaver several hours after death. My own experience is that the machine gives reproducible results provided it is used carefully. For example, I have never failed to find a pair of points at the back of the head, almost but not quite corresponding in position to GB20. Constant points can also be found on the ear and probably elsewhere. Sometimes the passage of the electrical current through them produces a pricking sensation.

Other kinds of point can also be detected with the Neurometer. Areas of decreased impedance can be found on the back, though they are not as sharply demarcated as those on the ear or GB20. There seems to be a tendency for these back areas to become more obvious when there are active triggers. However, detecting them doesn't add any useful information to that obtained by simple manual palpation.

The practical use of even the best point detection machines is in my opinion small. At most they indicate sites on the skin where there is a change in resistance, but in most cases one is interested, not in the skin, but in trigger points or ATAs lying at some distance beneath the skin. I find it much simpler and more effective to use my fingers to look for such areas than to spend time attempting to do so electrically.

Conclusions

I don't find any real advantage in the use of electrical apparatus of any kind in acupuncture, either for diagnosis or for treatment. I emphasize that this isn't because of any objection on my part to technology as such. On the contrary, I enjoy using computers and am by no means a Luddite temperamentally. During my time at the Royal London Homeopathic Hospital I obtained quite a lot of electrical machinery of different kinds and experimented with it, but I was unimpressed. I now think that acupuncture is a simple manual technique, and the simpler it's kept, the better. Your fingers are better tools for detecting triggers than any electrical detector, and brief manual stimulation of the needles is all you need to get the maximum therapeutic response.

References

Baldry P. (1998) Laser therapy. In: *Medical Acupuncture: a Western scientific approach* (eds Filshie J. & White A.), pp.193–201. Churchill Livingstone, Edinburgh.

Brown M.L. *et al.* (1974) Acupuncture loci: techniques for location. *American Journal of Chinese Medicine*, 2: 64–74.

Needham J. & Gwei-Djen L. (1980) *Celestial Lancets: A history and rationale of acupuncture and moxa*, pp. 187–8. Cambridge University Press, Cambridge.

Reichmanis M.A.A. & Becker R.D. (1976) DC skin conductance variation at acupuncture loci. *American Journal of Chinese Medicine*, 4: 69–72.

Thompson J.W. (1998) Transcutaneous electrical nerve stimulation (TENS). In: *Medical Acupuncture: a Western scientific approach* (eds Filshie J. & White A.), pp. 177–92. Churchill Livingstone, Edinburgh.

Wall P. (1999) *Pain: the science of suffering*. Weidenfeld & Nicolson, London.

White A. (1998) Electroacupuncture and acupuncture analgesia. In: *Medical Acupuncture: a Western scientific approach* (eds Filshie J. & White A.), pp.153–76. Churchill Livingstone, Edinburgh.

Chapter 17

Ear acupuncture (auriculotherapy)

There are several methods of acupuncture based on the idea that the body is mirrored in miniature in various places. They are sometimes called systems of micro-acupuncture (not to be confused with Mann's use of the same term). The ear is the best known of these miniature acupuncture sites but there are others, including the scalp (Yamamoto Scalp Acupuncture) and the first metacarpal in the hand. I have suggested (in Part 1) that these systems can be thought of as neoclassical acupuncture, because they use some of the ideas of the classical system but apply them in a different way.

The story of ear acupuncture, at least in the West, begins with a French doctor, Paul Nogier, of Lyon (Kenyon, 1983). In the early 1950s Nogier was intrigued to find that some of his patients had apparently been cured of sciatica by a non-medical practitioner who had cauterized an area on their ears. On looking further into the matter he found that this form of treatment had been used in France during the nineteenth century but had largely died out by 1870. Intrigued, he began to search the ears of patients who were suffering from various kinds of pain. Eventually he concluded that the body is represented in the ear, upside down in a fetal position, with the head on the ear lobe and the spine on the ridge of the ear known as the anti-helix. This recalls the motor and sensory homunculi in the cerebral cortex first described by Wilder Penfield. On this basis, Nogier developed a micro-system of acupuncture which he called auriculotherapy.

Nogier's idea was taken up by the Chinese, who claimed that there were ancient Chinese texts describing this method of treatment; they then produced their own charts, which were not identical with Nogier's, and which came back to the West. Thus we now have at least two sets of charts: Nogier's and the Chinese charts, the latter probably based to a greater or lesser extent on Nogier's though not identical with them.

Few attempts have been made to investigate Nogier's claims objectively. Filshie and White (1998) were unable to include a chapter on auricular therapy in their book on medical acupuncture: 'Despite two valiant attempts by well-known experts, there simply are not enough scientific data to give sufficient substance to the text.' Nevertheless, Oleson and colleagues (1980) at UCLA School of Medicine found some evidence to support the idea that there is a connection between the auricle and earlier health problems. Forty patients suffering from musculoskeletal pain in various parts of their body were tested. They were draped with a sheet to conceal any visible physical problems and then a doctor who knew nothing about their illness examined their ears for areas of increased electrical conductance or tenderness. A correct identification was obtained in 361 of 480 individual comparisons (75.2 per cent). There were 12.9 per cent false-positive points and 11.9 per cent false-negative points.

This is an interesting study and its results are striking enough to prevent one from dismissing the idea of an ear representation of the body out of hand. The ear does have an exceptionally complicated nerve supply (greater auricular branch of the cervical plexus, lesser occipital nerve, auricular branch of the vagus, and auriculotemporal nerve). It is therefore at least conceivable that the ear is connected with centres in several different parts of the brain and thus with remote parts of the body. But while this fact – if it is a fact – would certainly be very interesting for neuroanatomists, would it have any practical importance? Oleson and coworkers (1980) think that it would not help much in diagnosis, since generally it would be easier simply to ask patients where they felt pain. However it could be useful for unconscious patients or children, and they also found some patients who, when told of the findings of the ear examination, suddenly remembered previously forgotten pains or problems in the relevant area, and they therefore suggest that ear examination could be useful in the general assessment of a patient.

The main claim made on behalf of Nogier's work, however, is that it provides an effective method of treatment. When a reactive point is found in the ear this is treated by needling, sometimes with electrical stimulation of the needle. Moreover, Nogier moved on considerably from the simple initial method of examining the ear for tender points. He designed a number of electrical instruments for detecting points in the ear, and in 1966 he described the 'auricular cardiac reflex': that is, there are said to be changes in the amplitude of the radial pulse in response to various stimuli. Perhaps the most startling of his ideas concerns the use of coloured filters which are applied to the skin of the ear; different colours are said to have various effects on the pulse.

Needling of the ear should be done carefully. A fine needle (15 mm) should be used and it should not be inserted into the cartilage, but only just through the skin. The treatment is quite painful.

One problem with ear acupuncture, which is admitted even by its advocates, is that relief of pain often lasts only a short time. Semipermanent needles are therefore sometimes inserted in the ear and left *in situ* for about 7 days in an attempt to prolong the effect. As noted in Part 2, there is a risk of local infection and of bacterial endocarditis if this is done, so the technique should be used only in exceptional circumstances, on inpatients (see below). If prolonged stimulation is thought desirable, small balls that don't penetrate the skin are available.

I have experimented at times with ear acupuncture and occasionally found good results; however, I was unable to convince myself that I was able to achieve anything using the ear that I couldn't also achieve using 'old-fashioned' manual body acupuncture. The principal exception to this statement was in a case of severe unexplained abdominal pain.

A patient was admitted to our hospital with severe unexplained abdominal pain, for which she had in the past had no fewer than thirteen laparotomies. She was receiving large doses of conventional morphine-type analgesics and had also had every imaginable form of complementary treatment, including homeopathy, acupuncture, and TENS. She was writhing in pain and vomiting. In desperation, I looked at her ear, and found, at the margin of the ear on the same side as the pain, a small very tender area. This was not at a site linked to the abdomen in Nogier's charts. I needled this site as accurately as I could (it was very small, perhaps a millimetre or two in diameter), and the result was immediate lessening of her pain. We therefore kept a needle in place and connected it to a TENS machine to give continuous stimulation. The pain disappeared over the next few days and the patient was able to leave hospital. She was then well for about 6 months, after which she had a recurrence of the pain and was readmitted. This cycle of events was repeated at approximately 6-monthly intervals over a number of years. On each occasion she was admitted to hospital and the ear acupuncture was repeated. The treatment worked each time, although as the years went by she seemed to become habituated to some extent: the treatment took longer to act and the relief in between treatments was less complete than it had been at first.

Subsequently I looked for a similar tender area in the ears of other patients with abdominal pain but didn't find it. What was striking in the case of the original patient was the small size of the sensitive area in the ear and the accuracy with which she was able to identify it; she could always say whether the needle was in the right place.

Treatment of addiction, smoking, and overeating

There has been considerable interest in the use of acupuncture, particularly electro-acupuncture, to help in the management of patients addicted to drugs, alcohol, tobacco, or overeating. The ear is the site most often needled for this purpose. There is a site known as Shenmen near the upper pole of the auricle which is commonly used, and other sites are those lower down and supposed to be associated with the stomach (for obesity) or the lung (for smoking). There are many variations. Sometimes these sites are stimulated either manually or electrically during clinic sessions, and sometimes stud needles are inserted for a week or more at a time, the patient being instructed to press the needle (covered with an adhesive plaster) whenever the urge to eat or smoke comes on. For reasons discussed in Chapter 4, leaving needles *in situ* for prolonged periods is undesirable and it is safer to use balls fixed in place for local pressure.

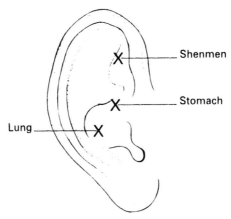

Sites in auricle used for treating smoking and obesity

The rationale for using acupuncture in this way is usually said to be that it causes the release of endogenous opioids. A recent review (Marcus, 1998) concluded that, although some early studies were encouraging, there is not yet a sufficient body of valid evidence to confirm specific effects from acupuncture, especially in the management of alcohol dependence, smoking, and overeating. The treatment of these dysfunctions is extremely complex and involves the management of a wide range of social and psychological factors, so that it is almost impossible to disentangle the role, if any, that acupuncture may have. If it does have any value, it's likely to be in alleviating discomfort during the initial period of withdrawal and perhaps by augmenting the effect of suggestion by means of its placebo effect. I have not myself used acupuncture in this way.

References

Filshie J. & White A. (eds) (1998) *Medical Acupuncture: a western scientific approach.* Churchill Livingstone, Edinburgh.

Kenyon J.N. (1983) *Modern Techniques of Acupuncture*, pp. 65 *et seq.* Thorson Publications, Wellingborough.

Marcus P. (1998) Acupuncture for the withdrawal of habituating substances. In: *Medical Acupuncture: a Western scientific approach* (eds Filshie J. & White A.), pp. 361–74. Churchill Livingstone, Edinburgh.

Oleson T.L., Kroening R.J. & Bressler D. (1980) An experimental evaluation of auricular diagnosis: the somatotopic mapping of musculoskeletal pain at ear acupuncture points. *Pain,* 8; 217–29.

Chapter 18

Self-treatment with acupuncture

From time to time, practitioners of acupuncture ask whether it is desirable for patients to do their own treatment. This suggestion sometimes elicits cries of horror, mainly from traditionalists who regard acupuncture as an esoteric affair requiring years of study before it can be practised adequately. This does not apply to my view of acupuncture, so the question is mainly one of safety. Considering that diabetic patients give themselves insulin injections daily or more frequently, and other classes of patients are also taught to inject themselves, I find it hard to understand why an intelligent patient can't be taught to insert a plain needle fairly superficially, perhaps only once a month. At any rate, I, in common with other acupuncture practitioners at our hospital and elsewhere, have taught a good number of patients to do their own acupuncture, and in many years no problems have arisen.

There are two main sets of circumstances in which self-acupuncture may be appropriate. Some patients have difficulty in attending for treatment regularly for one reason or another. Other patients suffer from disorders that respond quite well to acupuncture but only for short periods, sometimes for just a week or two. When I first started practising acupuncture I thought that if one gave such patients more frequent or even daily treatment for a time, perhaps as inpatients, there would then be a carry-over for some months after the intensive course. However, this never worked; the duration of any remission appears to be pretty well fixed for each patient, and this pattern of response is nearly always apparent after about six treatments or fewer. In such cases self-acupuncture seems like a good option.

Naturally, certain precautions have to be taken. Not every patient is happy about the idea of self-treatment, although a perhaps surprisingly large number are; if patients are reluctant it is sometimes possible to find a family member or a friend to do the treatment. The disorder for which the patient is being treated must have been shown to respond adequately in this instance. The patient (or other person who is to do the treatment) must be of reasonable intelligence. Finally, it is of course essential that the site to be needled is anatomically safe and easily accessible. In practice, I have most frequently used LR3 in this way, although other sites have been the target on occasion; for example, some patients with ulcerative colitis have been taught to do their own treatment by needling the lower abdomen, which is perfectly safe provided there is adequate subcutaneous tissue in this region. For self-acupuncture, patients are taught to use short (15 mm) needles, so as to reduce still further the risk of anatomical damage.

Having decided, after discussion with the patient, that this is the best plan to follow, I then make a slightly longer than usual appointment for the instruction to be given. The patient will already be familiar with the procedure, having had acupuncture several times previously, but on this occasion I repeat the treatment on one side, explaining what I am doing, and then the patient needles the opposite side under my supervision. If all goes well, as it nearly always does, the patient is told how to obtain a supply of needles. (The hospital pharmacy used to sell them for our patients.) The patient then goes home and carries out the treatment as prescribed for a few weeks. The frequency of needling varies according to the individual case; it might be as often as once a week, or it might be less frequent or might even be done on an occasional 'as required' basis. The patient is then seen again, and provided all is going well a further appointment is made for a few months ahead. After that it is often possible to discharge the patient.

It's important to make sure that there are suitable arrangements for disposing of used needles. When I first started teaching patients to treat themselves I used to tell them to put the needles in a tin or a jar with a top and bring them back to us for disposal. Nowadays some local authorities have arrangements in place for diabetics to dispose of used needles, or alternatively the local GP centre may be willing to take the needles.

Patients are told that they are able to telephone for advice at any time, although in practice they hardly ever feel the need to do this. They are also told not to change the site of needling without advice from us and to let us know if the symptoms change or the acupuncture ceases to be effective. I think it is essential to give them a leaflet (see below) summarizing all the points they have been told about. This leaflet mentions all the possible complications that might occur, including bleeding, infection, and broken needles, although it is emphasized that, apart from slight bleeding, these things are very unlikely to happen.

Experience with self-acupuncture has been good. Patients generally find it to be effective, although in some cases they report that it is not as effective as when they have acupuncture in the clinic, and they therefore like to come in for an occasional 'top-up'. This suggests either that they do the acupuncture less skilfully than we or, alternatively and more probably, that there is an element of placebo in the response in these cases and that having acupuncture in the clinic is more effective for that reason.

The following instructions and information may be given to patients.

Instructions for self-acupuncture

- Wash your hands in the usual way.
- Remove the needle from its envelope without bending it. (If you do bend it, discard it and use a fresh one.) Hold it in one hand (the right if you are right-handed).
- Stretch the skin with the other hand.
- Rest the tip of the needle against the skin.
- Press the needle quickly right through the skin, without hesitating.
- If necessary, push the needle more until it has gone in about a quarter of an inch (6 mm).
- Twist the needle gently a few times in both directions for 10–20 seconds.
- Withdraw the needle.
- Dispose of the needle safely.

Possible problems

- A small drop of blood appears when you remove the needle. Remedy: Wipe it away with a clean tissue and press the site gently for a minute or so. If the site you needled was your foot, keep the leg up until the bleeding has stopped.
- A small 'bump' appears when the needle is removed. Remedy: Press and flatten it gently with a tissue for a minute or two.
- Needle breakage (extremely unlikely). Remedy: Try to pull the end out with a pair of clean tweezers or similar implement. If this fails, consult your doctor or a hospital casualty department.
- Infection (extremely unlikely): The acupuncture site becomes red, hot and swollen, and/or red streaks appear running up the limb. Remedy: consult your doctor or a hospital casualty department.

Important notes

If any difficulty due to acupuncture occurs, please feel free to telephone this hospital to ask for advice. Ask to speak either to the doctor who treated you or to the doctor on duty.

Please follow the instructions given to you exactly, especially as regards frequency of treatment and site(s) of needle insertion. Do not change these without consulting the doctor. If at any time the treatment ceases to be effective, ask the hospital to give you a fresh outpatient appointment.

Self-treatment without needles: 'acupressure'

An alternative to self-treatment with needles is to use simple finger pressure over trigger points. This is often called 'acupressure': an unfortunate term, which really means 'pressure with needles'. It is possible to inactivate trigger points temporarily in this way, but the pain alleviation is fairly short-lived. Another disadvantage of this form of treatment is that the pressure may need to be fairly firm and sustained if it is to work, and this is often more painful than inserting the needle. However, it does offer a partial solution for patients who are very afraid of being needled.

Chapter 19

Training and accreditation

Although the techniques used in modern acupuncture are mostly simple, it would be difficult or impossible, and certainly undesirable, to learn them just from a book, so the first step in becoming an acupuncture practitioner is normally to attend a suitable training course. Quite a few courses in modern acupuncture for health professionals now exist. Although the organizational details will naturally vary from course to course, there is general agreement about the basic requirements. Courses should include a brief outline of the traditional system, in order to let students understand how traditional and modern acupuncture differ from each other, and also because it is at present impossible to be 'literate' in acupuncture without an understanding of the essentials of the traditional version. There will also be an account of the neurophysiological basis for acupuncture, to show how it can be understood in modern terms. Most of the course, however, should be practical, and should provide students with plenty of opportunity to try out the treatments on one another, so that they know what acupuncture feels like both as patient and as practitioner. This is best done with a mixture of informal talks and practical sessions.

Good needle technique is important for acupuncture: the effectiveness of the treatment depends in part on the ability to insert the needles skilfully and relatively painlessly as mentioned in Chapter 5, Principles of treatment. Students may begin by needling oranges, which is easy, and then repeat the exercise through a piece of thin card laid over the orange, which is more difficult. This doesn't mimic the sensation of needling human skin exactly but it is fairly similar, and it allows students to acquire the basic manipulative skills that are needed. Physiotherapists and osteopaths have generally not used needles previously and, although doctors are of course accustomed to this, the skills needed to manipulate the flexible needles used in acupuncture are different from those required for giving injections or taking blood samples.

The students next put some needles into one another, and the more adventurous often try needling themselves as well. This can be quite a testing experience for some, especially those whose clinical experience has not so far entailed the insertion of needles. At the end of a course for physiotherapists which I ran in Northern Ireland some years ago, one of the participants admitted to me afterwards that he had had to screw his courage up for 24 hours before attending and nearly turned tail at the last moment. However, most quickly begin to feel accustomed to the experience, both as needlers and needled.

Safety is, of course, the most important consideration of all. Students therefore are taught about this in detail and answer a safety questionnaire to make sure that they have understood the potential dangers of acupuncture. They also give a practical demonstration of their ability to needle vulnerable sites such as GB20, GB21, and CV17.

The knowledge and skill imparted in this first part of the training is common to all courses in modern acupuncture for health professionals. Differences in emphasis may emerge as the course moves on to consider the application of acupuncture to treat the various disorders; some tutors use the traditional terminology of 'points' to a greater or lesser extent, while others, including me, have developed their own descriptive schemes. This variation is not, in my view, a bad thing, since it shows that our understanding of acupuncture is still at an early stage. Indeed, it is probably an advantage for postgraduate students to attend more than one course, so that they get an idea of the range of possible approaches that exist.

Introductory courses generally concentrate on manual body acupuncture, but they should also provide a brief account of specialized forms of acupuncture such as auriculotherapy and the uses of electricity in acupuncture, though these are included mainly for information at this stage.

At the end of the course the students should be equipped with the essential knowledge they need to start using the treatment safely and effectively. They can then build on this progressively as their skills and confidence develop. The question of duration of training is, as we saw in the Introduction, a contentious matter. Traditionalists generally say that many hundreds of hours are needed in order to become competent in acupuncture, which is indeed true for the traditional version, especially when many of the students come from a non-clinical background. The British Acupuncture Council trains students over three years in part-time courses that include instruction in basic human sciences. The essentials of modern acupuncture, in contrast, can be grasped by most health professionals in the course of a weekend, though this is often followed by a second weekend in which the preliminary experience of using acupuncture is discussed and evaluated. What is then required is continuing practice in using the techniques and learning how to select suitable patients for treatment, all of which is an extension of the practitioners' existing skills rather than a radically new departure. This means that 'advanced acupuncture', which students sometimes ask about, doesn't really exist. The techniques themselves are nearly all simple: it's knowing when and how to apply them that is important. In other words, acupuncture, in common with other forms of treatment, depends critically on clinical judgement.

Of course, this statement shouldn't be taken to mean that a couple of weekends are enough to turn a novice into a fully competent acupuncturist. However, what is needed is not hours and hours of further instruction, but rather practice together with the opportunity to meet colleagues who are using acupuncture, to discuss successes and failures, and to obtain feedback from those who are more experienced. This can be achieved in various ways. One way, certainly, is to attend formal follow-up courses, and, as I have said, these have their place; but it can also be useful to meet in informal groups, to attend scientific meetings and lectures, to communicate via the Internet, and so on. Reading is helpful too, although its role should not be exaggerated, because acupuncture is above all a practical affair and there is no substitute for hands-on experience.

The novice should take every opportunity to use acupuncture. One quite common mistake is to treat mainly those patients who have failed to respond to the practitioner's usual forms of treatment. The right approach is to think of acupuncture first rather than last, and to try it whenever there is a reasonable indication for doing so and the patient is willing to have it. When acupuncture is carried out in the manner I have described, it isn't time-consuming and can be incorporated seamlessly into the rest of clinical practice. By using it frequently in a wide variety of circumstances the practitioner gets to know its strengths and its weaknesses and continues to build up the manual skills on which success depends.

Acupuncture societies and accreditation

Accreditation in acupuncture is increasingly becoming a hot topic today, though it is still at an early stage. The two main acupuncture associations for British health professionals are the British Medical Acupuncture Society (BMAS) for doctors and the Acupuncture Association of Chartered Physiotherapists (AACP) for physiotherapists; and both of these have accreditation schemes in place. Membership of the BMAS is open to all GMC-registered doctors but is not, in itself, evidence of any particular level of competence; indeed, members may not necessarily practise acupuncture but may merely be interested in the subject. However, the Society offers two levels of accreditation to its members. The Certificate of Basic Competence is awarded to doctors who have attended a recognized course, have submitted a certain number of cases for consideration, and have completed a safety questionnaire. The Certificate of Accreditation is for doctors who have been practising acupuncture for some years and who have submitted a larger number of cases, described in more detail than for the basic certificate. Re-accreditation is required every five years and is dependent on the provision of evidence to show that the practitioner has been keeping up to date with acupuncture.

The AACP is a Clinical Interest Group within the Chartered Society of Physiotherapists. Certificates issued to blood donors by registered members of the AACP are accepted as proof of safe practice by the National Blood Service. There are several grades of membership, with varying training requirements; Basic Membership is available to physiotherapists who attend an approved course which provides a minimum of 30 hours' training, after which they must maintain a minimum of 10 hours' training every two years in order to keep up their membership. Associate membership is open to other health professionals as well as physiotherapists, including osteopaths, chiropractors, and podiatrists with an interest in acupuncture. It is likely that these groups, too, will set up acupuncture societies within their own organizations in the future.

The question of accreditation is complex and is likely to change in various ways in the coming years. It is not at present compulsory for doctors or physiotherapists who practise acupuncture to be members of their respective acupuncture associations, although it is generally desirable that they should be. Not only does being a member help the practitioner to keep up to date with what is happening in acupuncture, but the more health professionals identify themselves with the treatment, the faster it will become accepted by their colleagues as a valid form of therapy and the more authoritative will those organizations be in negotiations with government about acupuncture regulation, which is certainly coming. These regulatory changes are part of the wider process by which unconventional treatments, such as acupuncture, are increasingly becoming accepted as adjuncts to conventional medicine. I touch on this question again in the next chapter.

Chapter 20

The future of acupuncture in the West

We live at a time of great changes for medicine, when advances in our knowledge of biology and genetics are beginning to transform dramatically the possibilities for treatment. Paradoxically, however, one of the most remarkable developments in the last quarter of the twentieth century has been the growth of interest in unconventional medicine. This is reflected in the names that have been applied to these unorthodox systems. First we had 'fringe medicine'; this has progressively metamorphosed into 'alternative medicine', 'complementary medicine', 'integrated medicine', and now 'complementary/alternative medicine' (CAM). These changes are supposed to indicate ever-increasing integration of the orthodox and the unorthodox. Not everyone, on either side of the divide, is enthusiastic about this. For some alternative practitioners, the whole point is to be different from conventional medicine, usually labelled pejoratively as 'allopathy'. Many conventional doctors, in contrast, still dismiss the whole of unorthodox medicine as superstition or worse, although the number of those who think in this way seems to be diminishing.

There have been two main consequences of the increase in public and professional interest in unconventional medicine. One has been a demand for evidence of effectiveness, which has come from the health authorities who are asked to pay for the treatment quite as much as from scientifically minded critics. The other is movement towards setting up regulatory bodies to supervise standards and training in order to protect the public. Both of these developments are likely to affect acupuncture as we move into the twenty-first century.

Evidence-based acupuncture?

In 1998 the Annual Representative Meeting of the British Medical Association passed a Resolution requesting the Board of Science and Education to look into the scientific basis and efficacy of acupuncture and the quality of training and competence of its practitioners. The Board's report appeared in 2000 and was broadly sympathetic to acupuncture; more so than two earlier reports published in 1986 and 1993. The report accepted that acupuncture seems to be useful for back and neck pain, osteoarthritis, headache, and nausea and vomiting. It found that acupuncture was ineffective for smoking cessation, weight loss, tinnitus, and asthma. It also made the important point that scientific evidence of effectiveness is not necessarily the same as cost-effectiveness; even if the value of a treatment can be partially or wholly ascribed to the placebo effect, it may still be useful in clinical practice and should not be ignored on that ground alone. However, the dangers of acupuncture were also pointed out in the report and this led to a number of recommendations about training.

The BMA report made the usual plea for more research. This is in danger of becoming a ritual incantation in such documents, but it does signal a real and serious lack. Medicine these days is expected to be 'evidence-based', and it has to be admitted that the evidence base for acupuncture is still fairly weak. There is a large amount of Chinese research material but this commands little respect in the West (Hayhoe, 1998). Even when it is available in translation, the norms of research that apply in China for traditional medicine are mostly very different from those prevailing in the West. Hardly any trials are randomized controlled trials. Most claim success rates that strike Western acupuncturists as improbably large – 100 per cent in many cases – and a recent review found no trial with a reported success rate lower than 87.5 per cent. Such claims excite scepticism in Western readers, but they really reflect a different way of describing the results, which tends to exaggerate the benefits. If lesser degrees of benefit are excluded, and only 'cure' or 'marked improvement' are accepted as indicating success, the response rate reduces to about 70 per cent, which is more reasonable. Most Chinese research in acupuncture is never translated, and even those articles that do appear in the West contain mistranslations of medical terms. For all these reasons, the Chinese literature is unlikely to have much impact on Western medical opinion in the foreseeable future.

Research in the West isn't without its problems either (Lewith & Vincent, 1998). Hitherto, many who have published papers on acupuncture have been inexperienced in research techniques. They have been working alone or in small hospital centres, with inadequate patient numbers, difficulty in finding suitable controls, and no statistical advice. University departments don't always show much interest in acupuncture research, and even when they do, the academics don't always know a great deal about acupuncture.

A recurrent difficulty attends the question of choosing a suitable control procedure. To the mildly interested onlooker with no particular interest in acupuncture it might seem that it would be enough to compare 'real' acupuncture with needling at non-acupuncture points, and a number of trials have used this method, which they call sham acupuncture. This approach is, at best, only suitable for the investigation of traditional acupuncture; it won't work for acupuncture which neglects or radically reinterprets the concept of 'points'. Fortunately, more researchers are now beginning to realize that 'sham' acupuncture is not equivalent to an inert placebo. An attempt has now been made, by Park and coworkers (1999) at the University of Exeter, to design a sham needle which doesn't pierce the skin but produces a sensation that patients would think was due to acupuncture. Evaluation of this instrument is now going on, and if it is successful it will be an advance, though it may not be without problems of its own. In view of such difficulties many researchers have concluded that placebo acupuncture is not a real possibility, and that a better idea is to compare acupuncture with other kinds of treatment.

Two fairly comprehensive reviews of acupuncture research appeared in the 1980s. Lewith and Machin (1983) reviewed 32 papers and concluded that the response rate is about 30 per cent for placebo, 50 per cent for 'sham' acupuncture, and 70 per cent for 'real' acupuncture. Most of the published trials, they believe, would not be capable of detecting differences of this order, hence one cannot necessarily conclude from these trials that acupuncture is merely a placebo treatment. They suggest that instead of comparing acupuncture and placebo it would be better to analyse the time for which a patient obtains relief from a given treatment.

Vincent and Richardson (1986) reviewed 40 studies. They, too, found serious shortcomings in most of them, but they concluded that there is good evidence for the short-term effectiveness of acupuncture in relieving a number of kinds of pain (mainly headache and backache but also some other painful disorders). They found the short-term response rate to be 50–80 per cent – higher, that is, than the expected placebo response rate of 30–35 per cent. The good initial response was not so well maintained, however, unless patients received booster treatments at intervals; this, of course, accords with what is found in ordinary clinical practice. No conclusions could be drawn about whether certain points are more effective than others.

Like Lewith and Machin, Vincent and Richardson were sceptical about the value of double-blind trials in acupuncture. They argued that single-blind trials are adequate 'provided efforts are made to monitor independently the impact of nonspecific effects and/or ensure that they do not vary between groups'. They also made a plea, which I would certainly endorse, for authors of research papers to give as much information as possible about what they actually did (number of sessions, duration and frequency of stimulation, whether de qi was sought, method of point selection and so forth).

In spite of the difficulties that attend the carrying out of good research in acupuncture, it's very important that it be done. Acupuncture has come and gone more than once in the West in the last couple of centuries, and there is no guarantee that it will not fall into disuse yet again. That would be a pity, for it has a valuable, if limited, contribution to make to medicine. At present it is more than half-way across the gulf that separates charlatanry from science in the minds of doctors, but if it is to complete the transition medical acupuncturists will have to produce evidence that it works.

An important review by Ezzo and colleagues (2000) was concerned with evidence for the effectiveness of acupuncture in the treatment of chronic pain. These authors had four aims: to summarize the effectiveness of acupuncture for chronic pain according to the type of control group; to see whether low-quality acupuncture trials are associated with positive outcomes; to see which features of the treatment are associated with positive results; and to identify areas of future research. Reports of trials in English were reviewed. They were included if they were randomized, had a comparison group, had a study population with pain longer than 3 months, used needles, and had a measurement of pain relief.

In all, 51 trials representing 2423 chronic pain patients were reviewed. Overall, 21 were positive, 3 negative, and 27 neutral. Most were small. Two-thirds were classed as low quality, and there was a significant trend for low quality to be associated with positive outcome. Trials in which equal therapeutic time was not spent with control and experimental groups tended to be positive. All these findings, of course, support the view of critics who dismiss acupuncture as ineffective.

Four types of control groups were used: waiting list, inert controls (sham TENS, sugar pills, placebo acupuncture), sham acupuncture, and active control (TENS). There was limited evidence that acupuncture is better than no treatment (waiting list); the evidence for the other kinds of control was inconclusive.

For me the most interesting finding was that so-called sham acupuncture was as effective as 'real' acupuncture but both were more effective than inert placebo. This, the authors say, suggests that so-called sham acupuncture may not be a true placebo but may have analgesic effects of its own. On the view of acupuncture that I have been advocating in this book, this finding is, of course, exactly what would be predicted; I don't believe that there is such a thing as sham acupuncture, but only more effective versus less effective needling.

An interesting finding is that six or more treatments were significantly associated with positive outcome even when the quality of the trials was taken into account. This suggests that repeated acupuncture has a cumulative effect, although other interpretations (chance, or patient 'investment' in the outcome) may also explain it. However, my own experience, which is in line with that of many others, is that the maximum effect may be achieved in considerably fewer than six treatments at times, so there should be no question of stipulating this number as an irreducible minimum; each patient needs to be assessed individually.

What can we expect from future research?

A little before the review by Ezzo and colleagues appeared, Ernst and White (1999) had also reviewed the available evidence for acupuncture and concluded that the only compelling evidence for efficacy was in back pain (but not neck pain), nausea, and dental pain, although in the last-mentioned the efficacy was possibly not great enough to make it clinically useful. Like all the other commentators, they emphasized the need for further research, and they also acknowledged the difficulty of finding suitable control procedures. And they identified four possible outcomes of such research.

Possibility 1 is that acupuncture might turn out to do more harm than good, in which case it should be abandoned. Possibility 2 is that it might be shown to be equivalent to sham acupuncture; both could then be used for their nonspecific effects, whether or not these required needling. (This seems to me to pose certain ethical difficulties regarding deception of patients.) Possibility 3 is that traditional Chinese acupuncture might be shown to be better than Western medical acupuncture (and better than sham acupuncture), in which case the traditional method should be taught and advocated. Possibility 4 is that Western medical acupuncture will prove to be better than traditional Chinese acupuncture, and better than sham acupuncture, for particular disorders. In that case, acupuncture should be taught and practised in a Western medical context and traditional acupuncture should become a subject for scholars and historians to study.

As will be apparent if you have read the rest of this book, my assumption is that Possibility 4 will prove to be the outcome of research. This is what my own experience suggests and I think the trend of research is in that direction, although it certainly hasn't arrived there yet, and I should not wish to exclude Possiblity 2 either.

Ernst and White make two comments in passing which seem to me to be important. One is that the response of any individual to acupuncture may vary from none to a maximum; this relates to the 'strong responder' phenomenon. The factors which determine this are not understood. An experienced acupuncturist can often, though not invariably, predict who is likely to respond well to acupuncture and who isn't, but at present this is largely an intuitive judgement. As a first step towards identifying the factors involved, it would be a good idea to design questionnaires to be given to patients before treatment to see if any common factors emerge.

The second comment they make is that psychological 'preparedness' may be crucial in predicting a response. I think this is correct. It is almost as if patients had a switch in their heads which had to be turned on in order for them to respond to acupuncture. It's important to understand that this isn't the same as belief. I have never found that prior belief in the value of the treatment is necessary, and indeed it's sometimes those who were most sceptical previously who do best. However, patients do have to be in what might be called therapy-receptive mode. Needles are often inserted into patients diagnostically, for example to take blood or to record electromyograms, but these procedures seldom seem to relieve symptoms, probably because the patients are not in the right mode at the time.

The role of suggestion in acupuncture is very hard to evaluate. We are often told that a major reason for the success of complementary medicine is that the therapist spends a long time with the patient, and asks a lot of individualizing questions about the patient's way of life, diet, emotions, and so forth. This is true, for example, of homeopathy, and it is also true of traditional Chinese acupuncture; Ernst and White make this point. However, it isn't true of the sort of acupuncture I practise, which is typically done quickly and makes use of conventional diagnostic methods. I have never gone out of my way to persuade patients that a good outcome is likely; I nearly always give them as accurate an assessment as I can of the chances of success. Furthermore, I have found the success rate with acupuncture in NHS practice and private practice is about the same, whereas in most forms of complementary medicine the results in private practice are better, presumably because of the increased placebo effect due to increased individual attention and a longer consultation time. For all these reasons, it may be that the role of suggestion in acupuncture is smaller than is sometimes supposed, although I certainly wouldn't wish to claim that it's unimportant. It would be difficult to deny that patients may be influenced by signals that therapists must give out unconsciously. As we saw Chapter 3, these signals are probably not merely verbal; the process of examining patients for trigger zones is in itself therapeutic to an extent. Such considerations make it difficult to assess what happens during acupuncture.

Looking to the future

If we assume for the moment that research will increasingly lead us in the direction of Ernst and White's Possibility 4, what will it mean for the future of acupuncture?

At present, many non-medical acupuncturists, and some medical ones too, seem to think of acupuncture as a specialty in its own right. This view pretty well inevitably leads towards an overemphasis on the complexity of acupuncture, which begins to look like a highly esoteric pursuit requiring many years of study and practice before the practitioner achieves the exalted status of an 'expert'. I don't myself believe that acupuncture, valuable though it is, should be accorded this degree of independent status. Even in ancient China, it was never the whole or even the main form of treatment, and I don't think it merits being considered as a specialty in the West.

Acupuncture is in some ways similar to the use of local anaesthesia. This is a fairly simple procedure that many doctors learn as part of their ordinary medical training, and use for performing minor surgery, suturing wounds, and so forth. Anaesthetists learn more elaborate versions of local anaesthesia, but this is part of their wider training as anaesthetists; no doctors call themselves specialists in local anaesthesia. Acupuncture, I think, should be viewed in very much the same light.

Another comparison might be with hypnosis. This, like acupuncture, is still a somewhat questionable treatment in the mind of many doctors, but it is used by some general practitioners and also by some psychiatrists, dentists, and others; there is a Society of Medical and Dental Hypnosis. However, probably none of these practitioners would call themselves a specialist hypnotist, and to do so would invite suspicions of charlatanry. Svengali isn't a medical role model.

There are many acupuncture practitioners, including me, who think that the subject should move away progressively from its roots in traditional Chinese ideas. I see the future of acupuncture as lying, not within CAM, but as a technical resource that will be used by a range of health professionals: doctors, physiotherapists, osteopaths, chiropractors, podiatrists, and any others who treat pain. Simple forms of acupuncture will be taught routinely to medical students, and as they progress in their careers after qualifying, some of them will elect to take their skills further and to use the techniques more extensively; those who go on to work in pain clinics or other specialized centres will use acupuncture to a still greater extent and will contribute to our understanding of how it works. Research will lead to progressively better ways of applying acupuncture in the relief of pain and possibly other disorders.

To some, no doubt, this will seem an unduly modest goal. Traditionalists, in particular, favour a much more radical position. They see acupuncture, as part of CAM, leading towards a considerable revision of how medicine is practised; there are even extremists who look forward to a replacement of conventional medicine by the alternatives. In spite of, or perhaps because of, an experience of CAM lasting a quarter of a century, I don't share this enthusiasm. Although I can understand, and sympathize with, many of the motives that drive so many people these days to seek the alternatives, I have no doubt that the future lies in science. Most of the so-called alternatives have little or nothing to offer beyond emotional support, which certainly has its value but is not enough. The physical methods of treatment, including acupuncture, have real effects, but most of them, again including acupuncture, come to us encumbered with large amounts of intellectual baggage. This will have to be shed before they become as useful as they are capable of being. I hope I have managed to make a modest contribution to that process in writing this book.

References

Ernst E. & White A. (1999) Conclusion. In: *Acupuncture: a scientific appraisal* (eds Ernst E. & White A.). Butterworth-Heinemann, Oxford.

Ezzo J. *et al.* (2000) Is acupuncture effective for the treatment of chronic pain? A systematic review. *Pain,* 86; 217–25.

Hayhoe S. (1998) The future. In: *Medical Acupuncture: a Western scientific approach* (eds Filshie J. & White A.). Churchill Livingstone, Edinburgh.

Lewith G.T. & Machin D. (1983) On the evaluation of the clinical effects of acupuncture. *Pain,* 16; 111–27.

Lewith G.T. & Vincent C.A. (1998) The clinical evaluation of acupuncture. In: *Medical acupuncture: a Western scientific approach* (eds Filshie J. & White A.), pp. 205–24. Churchill Livingstone, Edinburgh.

Park J., White A., Lee H. & Ernst E. (1999) Development of a new sham needle. *Acupuncture in Medicine,* 17; 110–12.

Vincent C.A. & Richardson P.H. (1986) The evaluation of therapeutic acupuncture concepts and methods. *Pain,* 24; 1–13, 15–24.

Further reading

Many of the chapters in this book contain a list of references that will provide suggestions for further reading, but here I offer some comments on certain books and journals which I have found to be particularly useful, though it is, I should emphasize, a purely personal selection.

Traditional Chinese medicine and acupuncture

Kaptchuk T.J. (1983) *Chinese Medicine: the web that has no weaver.* Hutchinson Publishing Group, London.

A very readable and authoritative account of the traditional system, from a Westerner who lived in China and really immersed himself in the traditional system. This is probably the best introduction to the subject for people who know nothing at all about it.

Needham J. & Gwei-Djen L. (1980) *Celestial Lancets: a history and rationale of acupuncture and moxa.* Cambridge University Press, Cambridge.

Needham was a Cambridge scientist and academic who, with Chinese colleagues, spent many years studying and writing about Chinese science and technology. This book explores the history of traditional acupuncture in China and also looks at its impact on the West. Essential reading for anyone wishing to explore the traditional system in depth. See also the following for other material of indirect relevance.

Needham J. *Science and Civilization in China* (several volumes now published; abridged versions also available).

Not directly relevant to acupuncture but contains a wealth of fascinating information about the way Chinese thought developed and how it differs from its Western counterpart.

Nguyen Duc Hiep. *Dictionary of Acupuncture and Moxibustion*. Thorsons.

A useful pocketbook listing the channels and points, with translations of the names. Handy for reference.

Kuriyama S. (1999) *The Expressiveness of the Body and the Divergence of Greek and Chinese Medicine*. Zone Books, New York.

A fascinating discussion of the way the ancient Greeks and Chinese viewed the body. Much new material and a valuable corrective to simplistic views of traditional acupuncture.

Modern acupuncture

Mann F. (2000) *Reinventing Acupuncture: a new concept of ancient medicine* (2nd edition). Butterworth-Heinemann, Oxford.

An excellent, if very individualistic, approach to modern acupuncture. Highly recommended.

Baldry P.E. (1998) *Acupuncture, Trigger Points, and Musculoskeletal Pain* (second edition). Churchill Livingstone, Edinburgh.

A very good exposition of the trigger point version of modern acupuncture, including a good deal of the research background. Highly recommended.

Filshie J. & White A. (eds) (1998) *Medical Acupuncture*. Churchill Livingstone, Edinburgh.

The most up-to-date review of modern acupuncture. Not so much a textbook, more a collection of monographs on different aspects of the subject, but all the better for that because it emphasizes the lack of firm knowledge. Essential reading.

Travell J.G. & Simons D.G. (1983, 1992) *Myofascial Pain and Dysfunction: the trigger point manual*, Vols 1 and 2. Williams & Wilkins, Baltimore.

The essential source book for anyone wishing to know about trigger points in depth; all subsequent writers on trigger points draw on this work.

Ernst E. & White A. (eds) (1999) *Acupuncture: a scientific appraisal*. Butterworth-Heinemann, Oxford.

The most recent review of research in acupuncture; highly recommended.

Melzack R. & Wall P. (1992) *The Challenge of Pain* (revised edition); Penguin Books, Harmondsworth.

An excellent account of the modern understanding of pain mechanisms. Although apparently intended for non-professional readers, it goes into considerable detail and contains a lot of information that would interest the practising acupuncturist.

Wall P. (2000) *Pain: the science of suffering*. Weidenfeld & Nicolson, London.

A more 'popular' book than the earlier one written in collaboration with R. Melzack, but still of interest as giving the latest thoughts of one of the foremost researchers on pain.

Journals

There are few good acupuncture journals, largely because there is little good research on acupuncture and what there is tends nowadays to appear in mainstream medical journals. Most acupuncture journals are little more than newsletters. The principal exception to this is *Acupuncture in Medicine*, published twice yearly by the BMAS and now referenced on *Medline*. Material relevant to acupuncture can be found in other journals not directly connected with acupuncture, notably *Pain*, and sometimes also in the *British Medical Journal*, *Lancet*, *New England Journal of Medicine*, *JAMA*, and other general medical resources.

The Internet

There is of course a vast amount about acupuncture on the Internet, much of it of dubious quality. A useful resource, with links to hundreds of other sites, is Dr Karanik's page:

http://users.med.auth.gr/~karanik/english/main.htm

The BMAS web page is:

http://www.medical-acupuncture.co.uk/

My own acupuncture webpage is:

http://www.acampbell.org.uk/acupuncture/

Index

(Page numbers in italic refer to illustrations and tables)

CL

615.
892
CAM

Printed in the United Kingdom
by Lightning Source UK Ltd.
118384UK00001B/256

9 780750 652421